Rudy's Blueprint
Volume 2

Rudy Blunce

ISBN: 1517007623
ISBN 13: 9781517007621

This book is dedicated to the original
My Dad Rudi B.

A Few Questions Answered

What Is This Book?

My first book was originally conceived as a guide to eating healthy and working out – two of the primary passions and driving forces of my life. I'd originally written a number of chapters – *which would eventually become, **Rudy's Blueprint*** – around this idea but they took on a life of their own that was impossible to ignore. Ultimately, I felt that my health and fitness ideas needed a separate home of their own and so, **Rudy's Blueprint-Volume 2**, was born.

So what are we going to accomplish here?

When you put this volume down, you'll know how to *lose weight easily, work-out* effectively, and *maintain a sustainable health regimen* that works best for YOU! In fact, I'm so excited to share my experience with you that I want you to be able to call this work, *"the Book"* (complete with air quotes) when you explain to your awestruck friends and family exactly how you lost the weight.

Now what makes my path different from any other weight loss or fitness book?

First off, I write and publish with 100% independence. I have no sponsors to shill for or products to push, no outside agendas to maintain or insider partners to please, and I feel absolutely no need to cater to the masses. I am *not* a struggling writer and my fulfilling day job keeps my bank account comfortably full before I even glance at any book sales.

As a consequence of this economic independence, if I feel my readers need some occasional tough love, I do not feel obliged to pull any punches. So let me state clearly that this book is *not for the faint hearted*!

If you're looking for a shoulder to cry on-

That ain't me.

If, however, you want a logical, realistic method of transforming from fat to lean in *3 months* and then to toned or even *ripped in 6 months*, then *that is me*.

That is this book!

Rudy's Blueprint-Volume 2 is not just about a basic diet and work-out plan. *It's about changing your behaviours and attitudes towards eating.* I believe that once you fully understand your eating processes, instead of just going along with what you've been doing since the day you were born, you will find it almost impossible to introduce foul, unhealthy garbage into your body. Eventually your body will simply and rapidly reject that foulness it once used to feed on.

We are the culmination of our habits and the hardest thing to change is a bad habit. If you're used to junk food before bedtime, of course you'll need to work to change. This book will show you how.

Perhaps you've read about people going through *out-of-body* experiences. Well, I want you to have an **In-Your-Body Experience.**

I want you to change your LIFE. Starting RIGHT NOW!

Who Am I?

First and foremost, *I'm a foodie.*

I love to eat, and I eat heaps of food!

I don't deprive myself because I love trying all the wonderful items on the menu and *I am never, ever, EVER hungry.* You will never be hungry either if you follow this book's simple guidelines. But we'll get to that later...this is about me.

I'm a 39-year old, happily married, I.T. project manager and father of two daughters who currently resides in Auckland, New Zealand (by way of New York, London, and Sydney).

I've lived most of my life eating horrendously, never considering or caring about what I was putting in me and certainly never seriously concerned about how it was affecting my body, mind or spirit.

I've been overweight. Wait, *did I write "overweight"? I meant **fat***! And not just fat but a heavy drinker and a pack-a-day smoker to boot.

How fat was I? Well, let me say that I've been fat enough at times to where my neck jiggled whenever I moved my head. Thankfully, no more. I found my way out and now I want to show you the way.

Now you might think that perhaps I'm some sort of self-loathing, hard core vegan type of person who compulsively counts calories and stockpiles misery. Let me assure you, I'm quite the opposite. *I love eating desserts.* Maybe you do too...

The only difference between me and someone grossly overweight and unhealthy is that I just *know when to eat them*, and how to stay disciplined enough to not have my just desserts leave any lasting effects on me. In fact once a week I splurge on the dessert menu with my wife and we usually eat anything and everything that we can find on it. Think of Chris Farley looking over the entire menu and saying, *"Yes, that will do."*

That being said, I do *not* have a degree in nutrition and I am *not* a qualified personal trainer.

I've never tried to do either because, in my mind, life is too short. Everything I'm sharing here has come *after* my formal schooling and the only degree I hold is in economics. The simple reason I'm in I.T. is because it pays heaps more than personal training and for a lot less work.

I generally prefer to work on the more logical, practical approach to eating and exercise, with plenty of common sense sprinkled in liberally. That is what my plan is based on.

So for the haters, I can't and won't try to stop you from throwing barbs and firing bullets from behind your keyboards. You can argue over my science and continue to present your side but you won't be able to argue over my results. And if this book makes anyone, anywhere reasonably question their eating habits or gets them into the gym, then it's done its job.

Suffice it to say, I'm a simple man, this is a simple plan and it will be easy when you get to learn it, know it and *live it* like I do.

What's The Plan?

Eating

One important aspect of my eating plan is that it allows you to eat as often as you like...as long as you're eating the delicious food I recommend here. In fact you'll almost certainly eat even more than you're eating now and the weight will still fly off.

Need more convincing? How about this:

1) There is **NO FASTING**.
2) There is **NO CLEANSING** or any other type of deprivation involved (except for processed sugar).
3) There is **No Need to Purchase** over-hyped weight-loss products in an attempt to "turn off" your appetite.

These other "plans" are simply and completely unsustainable. What *we will* practice here is not only sustainable but will insure that ***you will eat yourself thin!***

People who are flexible with their diet are more likely to stay on a plan, as opposed to those who rigidly strain to control their food 100% of the time with little to no pleasure allowed. So please realize that you'll live more than a little when you're becoming the new you that I prescribe. If we go hard for 6 days and then eat what we want on the 7th (preferably earlier in the day), it will be *all good all the time*.

As to what we should eat, we cannot and *must not*, in my opinion, cut carbs completely from our diet because our brain needs them to function properly. Similarly, we cannot cut fat completely from our diet either. We need it to function and to absorb vitamins. When we cut one of these, the body tries to overcompensate by craving the other. This is natural.

I'm happy even to go on record and state clearly that no one should trust in anything that has the words- *fat-free, low-fat or sugar-free-* on the label.

And the only real meaning of, *"Zero calories",* is that the FDA will allow the marketer to claim, "Zero", because the calories are less than the amount the report required. Please don't get it twisted- *The only drink with zero calories is water.*

Appearance

In my life I usually see fat people as fit people trapped inside of bad habits only because they can't figure out how to transform. Caterpillars stuck in the chrysalis and needing that extra kick to break free. I picture them saying to anyone fit:

"Get me out of here!"

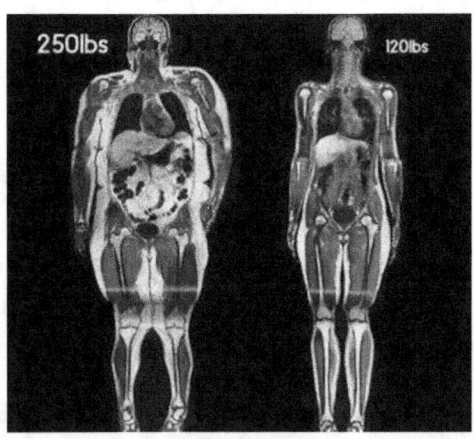

This is the reason I'm sharing my story and my methods. I believe that too many of us have surrendered to rationalization, convincing ourselves that it's "OK" to carry around extra, unnecessary, unhealthy weight. If you happen to be one of those rationalisers but actually believe that you're still eating right, this book can show you a truth that requires no such self-deception because I know this-

All that fit people are really doing to achieve fitness is eating better than fat people!

This path is not, however, exclusively for overweight people.

It's also for people who perhaps are already training, but aren't seeing the results that they'd like to see anymore. One of the most frustrating things is thinking that you are eating right and being good, and still not seeing good returns. We all know the popular definition of insanity: "Doing the same thing over and over and expecting different results." So let's all quit the craziness and face up to the facts.

If you want to look different, you need to eat and act differently!

Exercise

As far as the training portions of this book go, I will tell you what nutritionists and personal trainers don't want you to know. Maybe over the course of your adult life you've paid a small fortune for unsustainable plans and unrealistic goals. You have this book now and if you follow my path then you're good to go!

Following this path does require one thing: ***You have to be mentally strong before you can become physically strong.*** But don't worry, I'll teach you that as well.

Basically, your one and only body needs to become your one and only pastime. You may in fact need some new ideas and new directions to get past a plateau in your training. You may just need a kick in the ass.

Too many of us are stymied by those all too common trouble spots- How to get rid of my love handles, the cottage cheese on my legs, my beer belly, etc. *And etc.*

Well, this book will tell you exactly how to conquer these trouble spots but let me tell you right now –

It ain't gonna happen in any Spin class! You need to realize that your mind – *not your body* – is what's currently holding you back.

So let's talk about your mind a little and try a thought experiment. Imagine you woke up one morning and discovered that you have a 'god body'. You have the body you know you can have if you try. You are lean, as muscular as you want to be, and healthy. Now think about what you would need to do to maintain this body. What would need to change? Would you still eat crap (fast food, fried food, sugar, etc.) and expect your 'god body' to stay that way? Or would you need to think about your meals a bit more? Would you just ignore fitness and expect your 'god body' to keep its toned look? Or would you need to create a workout plan that maintains, or even improves, this cool new body of yours? What you think you would change to maintain your 'god body' is what you need to change to improve your real body...right now.

There is a simple, "biblical" rule to living on this path:

Muscle begets Muscle, and Fat begets Fat.

The path you choose to stay on will make it easier to stay on that path. So c'mon, let's take a new path – We're going to go places together.

1

The Proposition

Here is the clear cut, plain and simple, *Two-Step Deal.*

First, you'll absolutely require:

1) ***Three (3) full months of cooking for yourself* (work-outs optional) to lose the weight. We refer to this period as *THE SWITCH* and *THE WEEN.***

Then, after completion, you'll require:

2) **Another three (3) full months of cooking for yourself with prescribed work-outs if you want to get anywhere near firm, toned, or "in shape." This period is *THE BUY-IN* and *THE PUMP.***

Now let's take these one *step* at a time.

For the mathematically challenged among us the First Step means that if your goal is primarily *to lose weight only,* you'll only need three months to do it then ***BOOM***...you're ***DONE!***

This course will complete your *SWITCH and WEEN in 90 days*, which will be roughly *270 meals*, not including snacks. Now, can you spare yourself, your health and your one and only life for 90 days? Think of it as about as long as it takes to follow a great TV series but with a helluva lot better payback after you're finished.

Which brings me to the elusive, absolutely *magical percentage* of time spent working out that you'll need to do in order to lose the weight. Here is the percentage and it's easy to remember-

- ***It is 0%.***

That's right, you read that correctly.

You won't have to do one push up, one burpee or even one crunch to get lean. *What you are going to do is eat yourself lean.*

Then, and only then, do I suggest that you begin working out. You see one major misconception that is constantly sold to you is that working out is absolutely necessary to losing weight. I know that, in fact, *losing weight and gaining muscle are mutually exclusive – they can't happen at the same time.*

Of course personal trainers want you to work-out from Day One because, quite reasonably, it's their job and they'll get paid for their instructional, "motivational services." Now, don't get me wrong, intense training will speed up the metabolism of your stored fat. But it may lead to you becoming hungrier, which can lead to binge eating on all types of food (including junk) that your body will physically start to crave like a drug addict craves a fix. Perhaps you have some first-hand experience with this result which we will discuss at length in an upcoming chapter.

Now, does *not working out* sound crazy to you? I've no doubt it does.

But please think about it a bit more abstractly.

- *Do you put a dirty plate into the dishwasher with heaps of left-over food on it?*

Or do you rinse the plate off first?

- *When you leave the shower, do you leave water on your body?*

Or do you wipe a bit of it off, to give the towel a break?

It's a lot easier to get the job done, when you clear away the obvious stuff.

Here's another example. I enjoy training with a weight vest but find it impossibly difficult to freely and effectively move in space when I'm wearing 45 pounds (20 kgs) around my chest – *and I'm in good shape!* An overweight person is essentially wearing a weight vest all the time. So why would they think that, after years of abusive, unhealthy eating, they can just start working out while carrying dangerous amounts of weight? Seems silly when you look at it that way. What's more, this excess weight puts a massive strain on a body that is simply not accustomed to work in the first place.

This is not only unsustainable but also downright dangerous!

Our goal with *the First Step* is to make any training-to-come (and it will come) much safer, much more practical and *much easier on yourself* by shedding all that extra weight and all the heavy loads *first!*

Our goal, however, is NOT to just eat and remain immobile for 3 months. You will move and keep moving, you will shop, you will cook, and *you will be active in a manner that will become sustainable for a lifetime!*

In addition, the *First Step* doesn't mean that you'll need to practice any rigorous diets or do any ridiculous cleanses where all you drink is kale juice. You won't need to eat veggies all day or become an "organic" freak, espousing the benefits of quinoa and stevia to your bored friends and co-workers. No.

What you will do instead is eat *single ingredient foods* like –

Steak, chicken, fish, eggs, veggies, beans, nuts and much, much more.

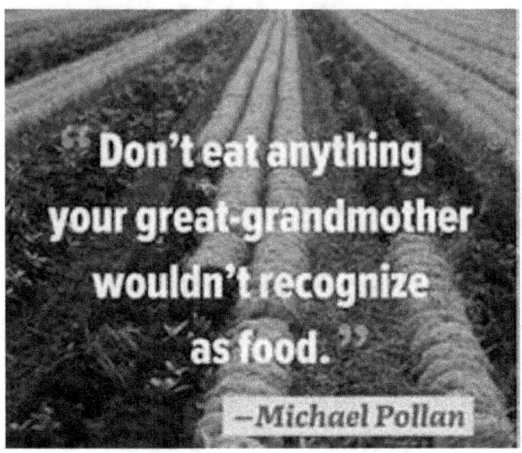

And you will never be hungry at any time. This *First Step* allows you to eat as much of the above as you want, and the weight will still fly off and I will explain the science behind this as well but to reiterate and reinforce: **You will eat yourself thin.**

So 90 days for the weight. Then another 90 days to get buff. Now why don't you see how we're doing after 90 days before you embark on the next 90? *Deal?*

The following chapters can have a great knock-on effect in your life.

This is what you will accomplish:

- *You'll eat healthy and lose weight.*
- *You'll start working out and building a toned body.*
- *Your muscles will allow you to eat more, and never be hungry.*
- *You'll gain confidence.*
- *You'll feel more comfortable making friends.*
- *You'll feel more confident at your job.*
- *You'll feel more comfortable finding a mate.*

If you think these things usually aren't directly related to one another, let me assure you that they were for me...and they will be for you too!

But before you think we're talking about Pie-in-the-Sky let me tell you one major downside to the plan-

You will be doing lots and lots of dishes!

Yet somehow, I think this is a small price to pay for the benefits to come.

So...are you still with me?

Then get that energy up...and **LET'S GO!**

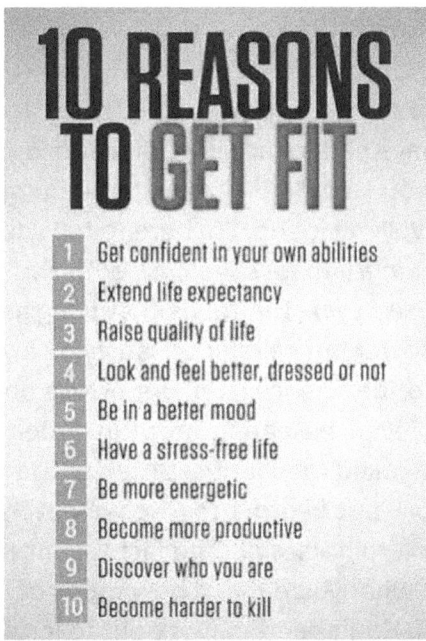

10 REASONS
TO GET FIT

1. Get confident in your own abilities
2. Extend life expectancy
3. Raise quality of life
4. Look and feel better, dressed or not
5. Be in a better mood
6. Have a stress-free life
7. Be more energetic
8. Become more productive
9. Discover who you are
10. Become harder to kill

2

Diet Lies that are Epic Fails

Before we get into the nuts & bolts of the plan, I'd like to take some time to review some common misconceptions that people have about healthy eating and some far too common misdirections that many of us have wasted our time and our health chasing. Think of this as some long overdue food for thought.

- *I have to eat less to lose weight* – The first and toughest hurdle most of us have had to face in our race to lose weight. How many times have you said, "If I'm going to be hungry all the time, why bother..."? Well my friend, I'm here to tell you that *you don't ever have to be hungry to lose weight!* With this plan *you absolutely will eat yourself thin*. The foods that I suggest in this book have no sticking power but will still be satisfying in every delicious way! We'll get into the science later, but please understand that some people may even be eating more in order to drop their extra weight. It's worked for countless friends and it will work for you.
- *I have to work-out in order to lose weight* – Nope, this common trope is absolute horseshit. The fact is your body weight is 100% the result of what you eat and how much of it stays on you. With this plan, you don't need to work-out to lose the weight because you're going to regulate your nutritional values and your intake. Of course, working out *is* a great step forward after you've lost weight but you don't need to start running, spinning, pilating, or joining gyms to lose weight. In fact, working out should not be synonymous with weight loss. It simply does not do nearly as much for you as refusing to eat shit. I often see fat people in strenuous work-out classes at the gym and I want to pull them aside to say, "You're wasting your time!" No class or work-out

routine will get you thin if you don't get your eating on point. If you are gung ho on working out, you need to channel that focus towards your eating for now.

- ***It's harder to keep weight off than to keep it on*** – I suppose the "harder" aspect here is subjective, but from my point of view, it's infinitely harder – both physically and economically -- to maintain a large amount of weight. First, you're paying for this excess weight physically by subjecting your frame to punishing damage on a daily basis. Second, you're (literally) paying for this excess weight with your hard-earned money because you constantly need to keep feeding the beast. When I look back at me at my unhealthiest, I now realize that I simply don't have it in me to eat enough to sustain 40-50 additional pounds anymore because I'd have to continually be eating crap food around the clock. Hey, right now I'd rather be doing more fun things with my life and you will too!

- ***I can eat crap because I work-out a lot*** – As they say in England, "Bollocks." I have a number of colleagues who work-out religiously (every weekday at lunch time) and they're no longer seeing any significant results after many months of disciplined effort. The main reason is because they think they've "built" their body perfectly by doing the same repetitive bench presses or squats and so now they can devour fast food or anything else and still remain fit. Nope.

Garbage In → Look Like Shit.

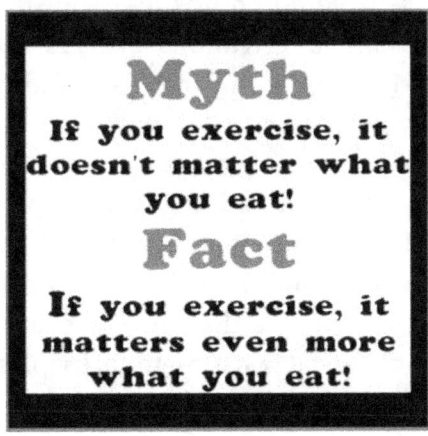

- ***I have to remove all fat or cholesterol or carbohydrates from my diet*** – Absolutely not. This is a popular misguided direction that people latch onto in order to seem serious or sound like they have a clue. You see when you attempt any carb-free diet, what you're actually doing is triggering the glycogen around your liver and your muscles into activation which is directly linked to water molecules. So, as a result, what you're effectively doing is losing a bit of water, which gives the *false positive* that your diet is "working" because you're temporarily losing a very small amount of weight. This "losing game", however, is entirely unsustainable as fat, cholesterol and carbs are and will remain absolutely vital to the overall health of your body. We'll get into each later, but you don't need to deprive yourself of any of these vital, healthy building blocks. The one exception is sugar, which *is* a type of carbohydrate. We'll get back to this later. What you will *need to do* is to remove any doubt as to where your food came from and how it was prepared.

- ***I have to fast or cleanse in order to lose weight*** – See above. Also see: *Rubbish.* What we all need to do is to *eat the proper foods in order to function properly!* By limiting yourself to one food, you'd miss out on the essential nutrients found in a wide variety of foods. Now I could and would make a lot more money (and many have) if I steered people into drinking all-celery juice or lemon detox diets but the fact is that these types of extreme deprivations are just not using common sense. There is nothing that any fatty faddy "cleanse" can do for you that your liver and kidneys don't do already. The liver and kidneys are your natural detoxers and cleansers and they will work perfectly fine if you give them the chance. If you're still considering juicing/cleansing then first seriously consider the nutritional information for *ANY* juice cleanse/diet because I guarantee you they'll either be low calories with high carbs plus sugar, or low fat with high carbs plus sugar. Those are both bad combinations for any reasonable attempt at losing weight and they're both terrible combinations for anyone trying to be even reasonably healthy. Don't waste your money or your life on these.

- **Eating healthy is too expensive** – If you try to eat exclusively organic and/or free range *everything*, or go to some esoteric speciality homeopathic stores for ingredients/supplements, then *yes*, eating healthy will be expensive. If, on the other hand, you simply *eat basic foods that have only a single ingredient*, you'll spend far less than when compared to consistently indulging on daily junk food and having sugar-packed treats at your daily disposal. I can attest to and assure you of this because I've been there! When you're cooking for yourself, instead of eating out or takeaways, you *will* save a bundle of cash following this path. You will also never go back to eating crap.

- **I can always find some place near work that serves healthy food** – In a perfect world, I would have a place near my work that served grilled chicken or salmon with fresh vegetables as a side. We live in a socialist/capitalist version of society however, and *these foods simply do not exploit profit.* Profit comes from mass producing low cost food and churning it out as quickly as possible, so if you think that you're doing your body a favour by eating a "healthy" sandwich (processed meat and bread) or sushi (processed rice), you're really not. That's akin to the ludicrous belief that "diet" soda is "better" for you than "regular" soda or that "gluten-free" cookies are better than "regular" cookies. Listen up because *processed shit is still **shit** no matter how it's packaged!* Any food products that advertise- low calories, low fat or reduced sugar are bullshit. **If it needs to say it then *you don't need to eat it!***

- **No one notices my weight because I carry it well. Besides, it's fun to be fat** – And here we have our very first tough love lesson because if you happen to be currently fat, then guess what... **We all notice it!** Think about how many people very politely avoid calling you fat now but, if you lost some pounds/kilos, they'd immediately and joyfully exclaim, "Wow, you've really lost a lot of weight!" Well, I've been told this and it always made me think. *"Geez, you've been biting your tongues this whole time?"*, as well as made me see my reality. It's exactly like being involved in a destructive relationship that all your friends hate and so they gratefully rejoice when you finally end it. But didn't you ever think, "Why didn't you guys tell me?" Well, my friend...WE'RE TELLING YOU! And we will all be more than happy to tell you that you look great after you lose the excess baggage. If you're currently rationalizing and unconvincingly convincing yourself that you're happy and jolly in a fat body then take a long look in the mirror buck naked. This is the *you* that everyone sees and imagines under your clothes, and this is what you can change anytime you're ready.

- **It's in my genes to be overweight** – A mammal's body is designed to store energy. Our animal cousins, the emperor penguins, store enough energy *as fat* to last them four months without eating while watching their eggs on their feet. So as a mammal, it is not surprising to be fat if you live a sedentary lifestyle. Your genes decide if your body has the ability to store fat in different areas of your body. Your lifestyle choices decide if you are just going to repeat your parent's eating habits. I'm telling you to break the mould. Don't play the hand that life dealt you. Make the dealer reshuffle!

> **It's not that diabetes, heart disease and obesity runs in your family. It's that no one runs in your family.**

- ***Everything that tastes good is bad for you while everything that tastes bad is good for you*** – Again, this is subjective but I find loads of healthy food to be delicious. Yes, I prefer to have a fine steak over a cheap hamburger and I'd rather have a perfectly cooked piece of fish over deep-fried fish-n-chips. Have faith in the plan because once you begin to eat healthy (and then keep eating healthy), foods that are processed, cheaply-manufactured, and ill-prepared will no longer satisfy your taste buds and will have a hard time working their way through the beautiful machine that is now your body. That's the place we want to be.

- ***All I really have to do to lose weight and keep it off is cut calories*** – It's time for our first science lesson: Calories are units of energy, and the amount of them you put into your body will either be used for energy, or stored as fat. In order to lose weight, you definitely need to consume fewer calories than what you're usually consuming. Conversely, the only way to *gain muscle* is to *eat more calories* than you usually do. Calories are important when trying to lose weight, but they *are not* the most important thing. Nature works in swings and roundabouts so if you create a caloric deficit, you may lose weight in the short term but your body will then crave a return to "normal" in a nutritional sense and if you're still eating shit food then you would not be improving your health simply by cutting calories. We'll do the maths later but a quick reference here is that both protein and carbs contain 4 calories per gram but 4 calories of protein is MUCH better than 4 calories of carbs. The common misconception is that the basic progression is to cut calories, lose weight and then achieve a balanced metabolism. In actual fact, the most effective method is to eat healthy in order to achieve a balanced metabolism, *which will then naturally reduce calories*, followed by losing weight near effortlessly. And once you add some muscle as well, the extraneous fat stays off. What we'll do here is change the quality of your food first. Later, we'll change the number of calories you consume.

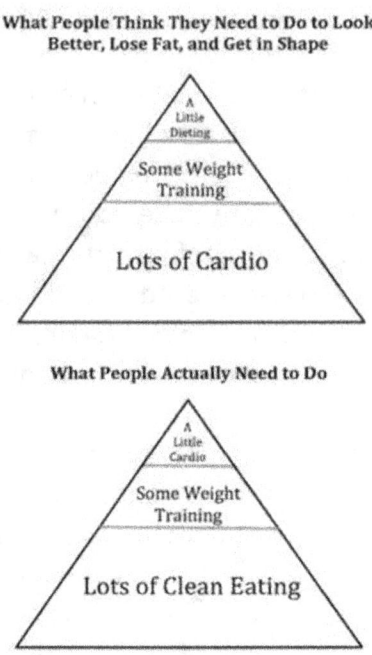

This is a fantastic site and another option for a further understanding of where people tend to go wrong in their process.

http://tinyurl.com/pchy6sw (This is the first of this book's hyperlinks. Obviously they're a bit easier to use if you're reading this digitally, but if not, no worries. I'd like for you to think of them as the cream of the crop of links to read on subjects. I've scoured the internet for you, and I'm hooking you up with the goods. Maybe they can be likened to a contemporary version of endnotes, and if you are interested in any of these topics, you can just quickly check them out online. And because I love ya so much, I've made them all tinyurls so they are easier to type.)

3

What Are We Doing When We Eat?

The Science of Digestion

OK boys and girls, let's do a physiology lesson here. Now don't bolt for the door just yet...

The reasons that all of us *"get hungry"* are directly related to our sensory intake of our environment (e.g. *hearing* bacon sizzle, *smelling* bacon fry, *seeing* bacon glisten), our gastrointestinal system (e.g. the peptide *grehlin* is secreted when the stomach is empty) and our metabolic signals (e.g. *catabolism*). As a delightful aside – *bacon is actually a part of our plan... **Woo-Hoo!***

Now I'll try to keep it brief, and feel free to skip to the **summary** in the end if you're absolutely science-challenged, but for those of you who appreciate *How Things Work,* please indulge in the following- ***10 Steps of Digestion.***

Now when we eat – when we literally make something in front of us, part of us – we first turn our food conveyor belt *On.*

Then-

1) **We begin breaking up food with our teeth and the enzymes in our saliva.**

2) **Our tongues taste the food then help to transfer it back towards our pharynx and into our esophagus.**

3) The mostly water-based saliva helps the esophagus to carry the food to our stomach, which is located behind our lower left rib cage (and not in the front or middle as most people think). The stomach releases enzymes and hydrochloric acid in its gastric acid.

4) The enzymes allow for protein and fat to be broken down into our body's building blocks, amino and fatty acids, respectively.

5) Hydrochloric acid kills microorganisms like bacteria.

6) The stomach then uses a process called peristalsis to churn and move the food (what is now called chyme) to the duodenum, which is the first part of the small intestine.

7) The duodenum has tubes linking to the pancreas, liver and gallbladder and releases enzymes that digest proteins, fats and sugars (carbohydrates).

8) The liver and gallbladder tube brings bile to the duodenum to help digest fat and the fat-soluble vitamins A, D, E and K. From this alone you can safely deduce that fat is vital in our diets, but I'll get more onto that later.

9) When fat, protein and carbohydrates are digested, the small intestine then takes the digested food and begins absorbing what it can use through its villi, and passing the rest through all roughly 23 feet (7 meters) of it. If only it took out the nutrients that helped you look good, and passed the fatty ones, it would be the perfect sieve but that is what you need to become. You need to be that perfect sieve by not allowing the foulness into your body.

10) Once nutrients are absorbed, they go into the bloodstream and eventually cleaned by the liver. (Please don't let my speeding through the process diminish how intricate and complicated

our bodies are and feel free to read more about their functions. There is so much beauty in what goes on inside of us.)

It is a wonderful process, and brings us to the crucial importance of the **liver** because this most vital organ is the unsung hero of the body.

Our liver is equally as important to us as our brain or heart. If we think of the brain as the processing chip of a computer and the heart as the power supply then the liver is the hard drive. If the brain is the CEO, and the heart is, let's say, the *Sales Team* of your body, then the liver would be the *Operations Department*, which is to say- *It doesn't get the credit it deserves, but would bring the entire business to a grinding halt if it ever went on strike.*

To take the Finance analogy further, I'll review a basic concept of settling financial trades.

When parties trade financial instruments with one another, they use a market so settlement of the trades is regulated and also so there is an *ease of use*. When there's a straight-through processing of trades, it means that there's no need for anyone to examine the trade for irregularities because the two sides are in agreement, and consequently the trades go through automatically. The funky trades are the ones that cause *exceptions* and need to be carefully examined and then stewarded through all the way to settlement. These more complex trades cause problems and cost money to sort out, which is usually more than the margin on the trade itself, so they often become, in effect, self-defeating losses. Well, it's the same for your body.

If you give it normal amounts of protein, fat and carbohydrates, it can straight-through process them with no problems leaving you looking and feeling great.

But if you punish it by eating tremendous amounts of carbs and fats, you make it work extremely hard to keep up, and you end up with the *exceptions* of body fat as well as additional physical maladies. You defeat yourself when you bite into that meat pie or giant, cheesy pizza or pasta dish. So why do anything to defeat yourself? Let's get back to the liver.

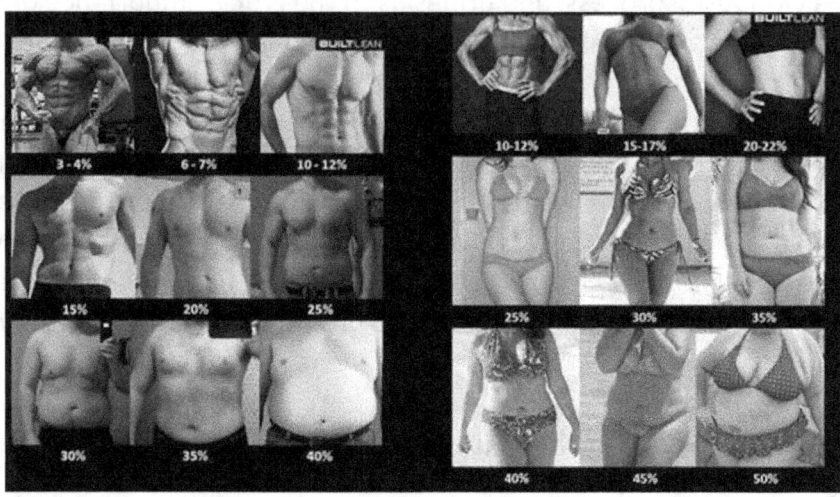

The liver stores vitamins, produces proteins, and cleans about 1.5 litres of blood every minute! Now all of us eat glucose in our food and glucose is a sugar that gives energy to all cells in our bodies, most importantly our brain and red blood cells. It's at the molecular level of every living thing in the world from bacteria all the way up to us humans. Now what the fantastic liver *also does* is convert glucose (sugar) into **glycogen**, which it stores for later use, if needed. This is how the liver regulates our bodies so that we don't end up with an overflow of glucose after every meal. When our blood sugar level drops, the liver converts the glycogen back into glucose and releases it back into our bloodstream. *This is called glycogenolysis* (don't shy away from the medical terms, there won't be any test later).

The liver works along with the pancreas to regulate the body. The pancreas secretes **insulin** when we eat any meal that has glucose, fatty acids and/or protein. When we eat lots of sugary food, insulin stimulates the body to absorb glucose from our blood. When the body has a large amount of glucose in its system, a larger amount of insulin needs to be secreted.

Now let's consider a common example.

When you eat a candy bar, or drink a soda, the glucose level in your blood will rapidly rise and the pancreas will then secrete a *mega amount* of insulin to keep the blood sugar levels from overflowing. This increase must, however, return to equilibrium. Consequently, in a few hours, the blood sugar levels will have to drop to *lower than normal* to compensate for the associated spike. That's why you may feel depressed after coming off a sugar high. This drop in blood sugar can also cause your body to release adrenaline which can lead to nervousness and anxiety. So the candy you ate to *make yourself feel better* has now evened out by making you feel like a hot mess.

Now, as the saying goes, you can only go to the well so many times. The problem with your body's fantastic digestive system is that it will continue to try to compensate for any poor eating habits until it begins to overcompensate. When it does that, the situation at the well becomes a lot more serious.

If you keep abusing the regulation of your insulin balance, your body will build up an insulin resistance. This means that your body will no longer *easily* absorb glucose. Instead, this gradually overcompensating insulin resistance will cause your body to hunger for more and more sugar to cover its energy usage. This will leave you feeling – *and likely behaving* – like a sugar fiend. Is this you? Do you crave sugar and not know why?

Of course the kicker is that if/when you abuse sugar and screw up your insulin balance (by eating refined carbs and foods lacking macronutrients), you'll end up in the rapidly degenerating cycle of physically craving more and more sugar to satisfy your now unbalanced insulin demands. It's definitely a slippery slope, and every slope gets slippery fast when you're a fatty.

But before you begin your slide – *or slide any further* – here is another big key to fat loss.

The fact is that your body ALWAYS requires energy to function. It's constantly working for you and, of course, it is always *On,* just like your brain. Your digestive system will command your body to perform glycogenolysis for fuel. Its go-to source for that fuel is glucose. If your body is *low on glucose,* the next source, and next line of defence, will be breaking down fats into glycerol and fatty acids. *This is called* **LIPOLYSIS (which has a follow up process called Ketosis)** and it is absolutely *KEY!*

If you limit the amount of sugar and refined carbs you put into your body, you'll inhibit glycogenolysis and, *as a direct consequence*, your body will rapidly turn to its fat stores as its default energy reservoir.

Many argue that by running, or working out, you're causing further lipolysis to occur but, in my opinion, you'll only be setting yourself up for increased sugar cravings. That's why I recommend that you should treat losing weight and gaining muscle as *two very separate tasks*. And for those who are attempting to "spot fix", you'll need lipolysis to occur and clear the way for your spot fix methods. You simply can't lose weight in one place without losing it all over first.

In Summary

This is how your body works:

- *Your blood has a small amount of glucose (blood sugar) in it that's constantly being used for energy. This will last for 20-30 minutes before the glucose needs to be replenished.*
- *Your body will always shift to any and every method in order to replenish its glucose to safe levels as your brain needs a steady amount of it to function.*
- *It will look to accomplish this first through the breakdown of carbohydrates which contain glucose bonded to other substances (Ex: if you're jonesing for potato chips between meals, your body is looking for an easy way to get glucose into the blood).*

- *Breaking down carbohydrates is much easier than the next available source which is your fat storage.*
- *Your body breaks down stored fat into glycerol and fatty acids in the process of **lipolysis**. The fatty acids can then be broken down directly for energy, or they can be used to produce glucose through a multi-step process called **gluconeogenesis** (where amino acids can also be used to make glucose).*
- *If no carbs are in your food, or body, the system will then look to turn **glycogen** (you have 360 calories to burn at any given time) into simple glucose molecules. This process is called **glycogenolysis**.*

What does this all mean?

It means that you need to fully realize and completely accept these **Four Simple Points:**

1) **Your body is going to call out to you every half-hour-on-the-hour in search of an available energy source.**

2) **It will then either use food, fat or muscle to create that energy.**

3) **If you're fat, you should allow your body to conveniently access your fat storage first by not eating refined carbohydrate foods.**

4) **Instead, you must eat high-protein and veggie foods for fuel. Doing so will make it easier for your body to access its fat stores for energy.**

So all in all, you'll need to look at your body as an exciting, real-life science experiment. Everything is energy. Everything has energy in it and your food is the same. It can be broken down to give you energy or it can very easily be stored as energy (fat). You must understand the effect of everything you're putting into your body and allow it to continue to break down fat instead of muscle for energy.

If I were overweight now, I'd eat high-protein and veggie-carbed meals with minimum sugar and I'd make *Optimum Nutrition 100% Whey Gold Standard* protein shakes my between meal snacks. This would allow me to feel satiated (instead of hungry) with lipolysis effectively burning my fat in the background.

You have the choice after reading this chapter and for the rest of your life to either:

- *Continue to introduce harmful garbage into your body or...*
- *Fuel up on healthy food that will allow your body to either burn fat or build muscle.*

You have the choice to either:

- *Dump scientifically-modified, preservative-filled food stuffed with an encyclopaedia of ingredients into yourself or...*
- *Get back to your more natural state with basic foods consisting of 1-2 ingredients max.*

You can keep pretending that you like being the way you are as you avoid all mirrors like a vampire and only remove your clothes when absolutely forced to (and even then only shamefully) or *you can do something about it*!

You can come to grips with the food you eat and the physical reactions it creates inside of you, and then truthfully, openly, unreservedly ask yourself if your food is helping or hurting you.

I want you to consciously think about what you're doing the next time you eat and – every time after that – continue to consciously appraise your diet.

"Why am I eating this?"

"Why do I do this?"

You don't need to be afraid of these questions anymore.

And just by the simple, straightforward method of making your body burn fat instead of sugar you're going to –

EAT YOURSELF THIN!

And I'm going to show you how...

4

Insulin – *Your Arch Frenemy*

Yes, it is.

And the reason insulin is such a key body secretion is because, to a great extent-

Insulin decides whether you will be fit or fat!

It's your frenemy because when you begin losing weight, you'll need to mute it. You'll need to learn to control it and then keep it from spiking. Now here's the tricky part because *when you begin adding/ gaining muscle*, you'll need to partner with it, you'll need to exploit it and you'll need to use it to your advantage by consciously spiking it around your work-out (we'll cover this in more detail in the *Working Out* section). So first let's talk about what insulin is and what it can do for you.

Insulin is a peptide hormone. You may remember from my first book that hormones regulate physiological and behavioural activities. In our human case, insulin regulates our metabolism. You've probably used the term metabolism in your life in the sense of, "He/she has a faster metabolism than me..." or "My metabolism slowed down after I turned 24...", but let's take a closer look.

Metabolism is divided into the two categories of **Catabolism** and **Anabolism**.

Catabolism is the destructive process that breaks down complex molecules into simpler ones in order to release energy (this could be fat or muscle).

Anabolism is the constructive process that builds complex molecules out of simple ones (again, fat or muscle) in our living tissue.

So which one does insulin fall under? Insulin is anabolic.

It will either help you to create adipose tissue – more commonly referred to as *fat*– or it will help you to create muscle by inducing your muscle cells to stockpile glucose, amino acids or creatine. We'll discuss the benefits of insulin in the second half of the book but, for now, let's just say that it is *not* your friend.

Instead, let's think of insulin as being a wise, welcome and always accommodating matchmaker. If you happen to be a hot piece of muscle and your body knows of some sexy amino acids looking for a good time...well then insulin will slide over and say, *"Let's get you two together."*

If you happen to be an unsavoury slab of fat and your body knows of a load of equally unsavoury sugar or refined carbs...well then insulin will slide over and say, *"This is the best you're gonna get, so deal with it."*

And that is how we get fat. Your frenemy insulin loves to hook up your fat cells with more fat.

This is a fantastic link explaining insulin and its effect on fat and muscle.

http://tinyurl.com/k8y9p85

The physiological reality is that your metabolism is either breaking or building your body all the time. You're either breaking down muscle (a big No-No) or fats (a big Yes-Yes) to use for energy or you're building fat stores or muscle. So with every bite you take, you have the opportunity to either *build fat* or *build muscle*. Start thinking of eating in that light and you're on your way down the path to good health.

You need to look at all of your food on a molecular level and ask how that food will affect you.

Using insulin to create fat is a cycle you must break.

But before we do that, let's talk about *why* we eat just...plain...crap!

5

It's Not Your Fault

I'm going to go out on a short limb here and say that you're not at fault if you're overweight. It's not your fault. And feel free to think of me as your fave late Robin Williams character giving you that big, strong hug while I'm telling you this truth that I've learned through my own tough experience. It's not your fault.

When we have crap choices to eat, we'll invariably choose crap. When I was living in New York, I was eating a massive bacon, egg, and cheese bagel every morning. My lunch and dinner choices were typically pizza, burgers and jumbo sandwiches occasionally broken up by Chinese take-out.

In London the jumbo sandwiches were called "Sarnies".

In Sydney they were called "Sangers".

And to make my global menu and everyday dietary intake even worse, all of these were cheap, convenient options that *required minimal effort to score*. Of course I was destined to have weight issues because I served up my appetite to the lowest bidder and I willingly placed my nutrition in the hands of others who weren't at all concerned with that life affirming concept. This was where I went wrong and then *willingly continued to self-destruct*. Now what I needed to do, and eventually did, was begin by preparing my own meals and taking control of what I was putting into my body on a daily basis. And *this is what you will need to do as well*.

If you're currently overweight, you're actually caught in a crazy vicious cycle of sugar abuse.

Whether you realize it or not, you've been physiologically and psychologically tricked into being fat. You've also built up such a resistance to your insulin regulation that your body now physically craves sugar as fuel – *much like a drug* – because your insulin is no longer effectively extracting the glucose from your blood. This is exactly how **fat begets fat**.

Once you start this chain of events, your addiction to sugar starts to grow exponentially. Your body will begin to crave more fuel, including sugar, to operate, or it will go into conservation mode, making you want to sleep more and/or exercise less. This is to insure that your existing energy levels at least get you through the day. Then, once you refuel, your food won't be completely used as energy because your body will seek to conserve it by creating more fat.

If you try to exercise in this unfit state, your body will crave even more food to sustain the energy needed to do so, kicking the vicious circle/ cycle into an even higher gear.

And this is why I believe that anyone currently overweight who attempts to work-out and eat right, sooner or later – and it's almost always *sooner* – will binge eat and undo all of the progress they thought they were making.

This is why I believe that like cigarettes, food can sometimes be a trigger:

1 candy bar = 1 cigarette

1 ice cream bar = 1 cigarette

1 bag of candy at the movies = 1 cigarette.

One cigarette begets the next cigarette physically and psychologically. That is why all smokers need to do is stop smoking that one cigarette. Now of course one cigarette won't kill anyone but all you need is one of these trigger foods to start a slow, painful process that will eventually do the job with nothing but misery along the way.

So let's attack the problem from a different angle. Let's get rid of the addiction and craving first!

We want to get you to a point where a candy bar in front of you is no trigger at all and you can easily say, "No thanks." With a smile on your face.

So is this a diet? **No.**

Am I going to tell you a special eating plan revolving around fasting? **No.**

Am I going to tell you to eat like a rabbit? **NO!**

Because the reality is that if you're overweight but really want to get into shape, or *back* into shape –

You don't need a diet. You need to change the way you look at food!

Food should be giving you the fuel you need to live. It doesn't need to be a contest every time you sit down for a meal. You don't always need to finish everything on your plate. I know this will be difficult for many – it was for me once too. Food should be eaten in *small-to-medium* sized portions that allow your body to properly digest it. You should be eating, and always seeking to eat, fresh ingredients. And you should be intimately aware of everything that goes into your meal and the one and only body you will ever have.

Let me tell you the honest truth: I once appreciated fast food. The operative word being *once*. If I eat fast food now, I get physically sick. I'm fine with this and much healthier because of it. You want to be eating fresh for so long that the very thought of ingesting anything processed

27

turns your stomach. Giving up fast food is like giving up cigarettes. Once it's in your past, you can't even imagine having another noxious ciggie, processed "burger" or deep-fried anything. You won't even think about it again, in any way.

I want you to get to the point where you think of the saying FOH (Fuck Outta Here) when you see shit food. Just dismiss it and feel good about saying no.

The Health Halo

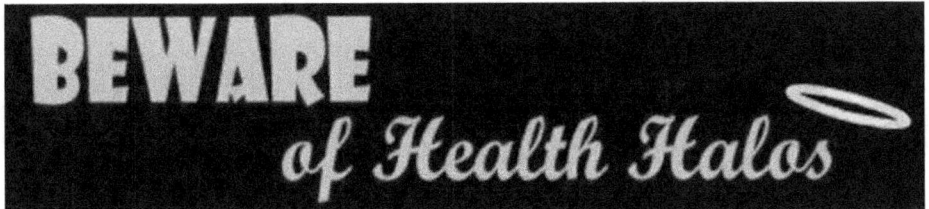

One thing that really grinds my gears is the wholly unwarranted trust that so many – as in *too many* – people put into "healthy" food. Malicious marketing tricks and tactics allow for corporations to claim and label their food as "healthy" when it clearly isn't. All with no consumer recourse. The entire food industry is dangerously unregulated thanks to career politicians who require corporate sponsorship to win endless elections. In the process of gaining these sponsorships and winning these elections, they treat regulations like the flu so the food industry can do what it wants. In this respect, the food industry is much like the shockingly corrupt banking industry in that our governments are simply too cosy, cowardly or just plain ineffective to stand up to them and do the right thing for everyone. Let me explain how this relates to you.

Corporations are created and live and breathe to maximize profits. They see opportunities in every fad or consumer shift and are always prepared to exploit these for their bottom line benefit. The latest fad is to advertise, through product labelling, their shitty processed food with deceptive buzzwords like, "heart healthy", "low-fat", fat-free" and "all natural". For example: If there's even a miniscule amount of fruit in a product, the label insures the consumer that it "contains fruit." Obviously they'd never label their garbage as, "high in fat" or "loaded with sugar" so instead the labels promote the erroneously safe, "high in fiber" or "contains calcium" to trick you into thinking you're helping yourself by eating them. When they are labelling a food, "fat free", it simply means that they've put more sugar in to make up for the missing taste. As there are no repercussions for companies putting incorrect nutritional facts on food, why would they ever tell the truth? By eating one-ingredient foods, you don't have to worry about nutritional facts or anyone lying to you.

Now, what do you think happens when most unhealthy, distracted consumers with bad habits believe a product is "healthy"?

Do they limit themselves to a single serving of that "healthy" fare, or do they believe they can, and even *should*, "load up" because it's "good" for them?

Do you remember *Sunny Delight?*

Do you remember it being marketed as the "healthier choice"? It was even sold in the chilled section of supermarkets as "real fruit juice" that required refrigeration to maintain its "freshness". Well...it wasn't healthier or the slightest bit fresh. It was putrid sugar water that had more sugar than most soft drinks. And the commercials encouraged parents to purchase it "for the kids" instead of the purple stuff? Of course this was blatant, egregious false advertising but there was no strictly legal recourse. You can't sue a company for making you fat as they can and will always claim, safely, that it was *your choice*. You need to see through the malicious marketing in this world and begin making smarter choices.

What con are they running? Cui bono?

You simply cannot afford to blindly trust marketed food targeted to deceive. You may likely know it already but allow me to make it even clearer.

You can get just as fat off **"healthy", "organic", "fat-free", "low sugar", "zero calorie"** food as you can off fast food garbage because that's exactly what all of it is! **"Sugar free"** simply means that a gigantic amount of *high-fructose corn syrup* is added instead, which is like switching ice cream for pizza and expecting different results.

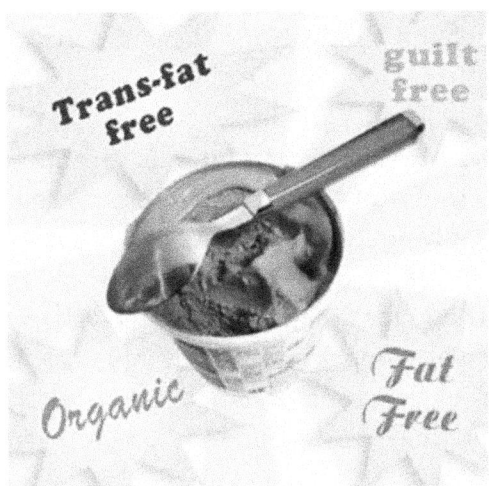

Using these deceptive, destructive marketing tactics, corporations have become deadly, insidious *Trojan Horses* designed to put you to sleep while they sneak even unhealthier, addictive food past your gob.

And if you turn a blind eye to what's really going on, this negligent, self-destructive behaviour then becomes ingrained. You'll feel safe, secure and even proud of yourself when you visit a "healthy" sandwich shop with your guard down and then proceed to order *the foot-long version* with the cookie too...and let's not forget the XL "diet" soda to wash all that "healthy" badness down!

This, my overweight friends, is insanity.

And you should always be on the lookout for the dangerous trade-offs every company uses to lure you into their consumer traps. They are almost always substituting damaging ingredients to add flavour and still keep their "healthy" label intact. Sugar is "gluten-free" ya know!

Even, or especially, at healthy food stores, the devil is "in the sauce" quite literally and often in everything else as well. What I do with my plan is to get you to *want to* eat fresh and free from sugar and all refined carbohydrates.

As much as I love all of the "4-Hour" instructional books, you should fully understand that you will never get a great body with only four hours of work a week...or even four hours a day! Your body is – and *must become – a 24-Hour Project*. You must become intimately aware of everything you're putting into it. There are no seven minute abs, or short cuts. You simply need to eat clean.

The food I eat now and for the majority of my waking hours is based on being fresh and always prepared by me. My typical daily menu consists of steak, chicken, eggs, heaps of veggies and fresh water. Does that sound ascetic or indulgent? Believe me, it's indulgent! And it's easier than you think.

Ultimately I believe that your body is the great leveller. It doesn't matter where you're from, what you do, what you drive, or how old you are because if you have a body you're proud of then you can always feel confident wherever you are. No one can or will tell you anything about dieting or working out if and when you're in good shape.

My plan works because this lifestyle shift in your eating habits works for everyone and at any age. You can feed your partner, your family and willing friends with this plan if you care about them, they care about themselves and everyone enjoys a delicious, healthy meal!

For you, losing the weight will be simple. Keeping it off will be even simpler. Getting yourself to take the first step is the hard part. Maybe your decision to read this book was a massive change to your mindset already. Once you get going down these tracks, I assure you that your train will keep picking up momentum. It is very easy to stay focused when your lunches are already cooked for you, and you're never hungry. Make smart and healthy choices and after a while you will no longer have to choose even. Throw in the working out later and the routine becomes your new normal, and then you don't need to think anymore, you just eat healthy and work-out hard. What starts happening is that you crave the intensity. You enjoy being good. You don't just work-out for 6 months and then go "let me get back to doing nothing and eating shit." And since you keep on going, your body keeps whittling down.

Being angry, disappointed, disgusted and depressed at yourself for looking fat, *without doing anything to make a change*, is like being mad at your playlist for replaying a song for the umpteenth time. You have to make the changes that you want to see. You have to do this for yourself and *NOW* is the time!

Once you get this plan into motion, you'll begin to see direct results and consequently you'll discover that changing your lifestyle is more reasonable than you ever imagined. I've been around the world, and I've seen – *and eaten* – some real culinary horror stories. Take for example, *the blooming onion* in the US, the *UK battered sausage and the Scotch egg,* and of course, the ubiquitous *French fries*. They're all slow forms of suicide and always reserved and ever available for those herds of heifers who've given up on eating right. Only *sheeple* eat fast food and it's past time for you to separate from the herd! I no longer can or will eat fast food. I certainly would never force my children to eat that food because I believe it's a passive form of child abuse.

Check this good video illustrating the grinding wheels being put in motion by fast food.

http://tinyurl.com/lco9q59

And here's a guy losing it over having to market the crap.

http://tinyurl.com/qj75vt4

The last time my wife fed the kids fast food two meals in a row, they got sick. You may doubt the correlation but it's enough for me. So let's all cut the crap out of our children's lives.

This site has additional illuminating insight on exactly what goes into fast food.

http://tinyurl.com/nkaesxj

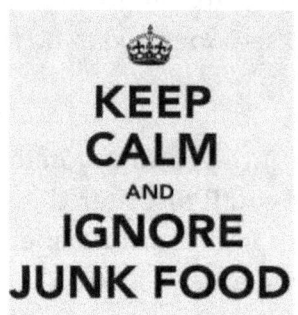

6

So Why Do We Eat Bad Food?

That's the big question, isn't it?

Don't worry. I've got some simple answers.

But first, in the interest of clarity, from this point forward I'm going to pleasantly refer to fast food, junk food and all processed food as, *"shit."*

A Simple mantra: If I eat shit, I will look like shit.

Say that to yourself before you eat anything that isn't beneficial to your health and well-being and if you happen to be reading this to lose weight...then you my friend, are eating *shit!*

It's not OK, but don't stress anymore because we've all been there.

From my own personal experience, and from the numerous experiences of all the diverse range of people I've interviewed for this book, I've found that the underlying reason and the most significant factor for most of the food decisions people make is **Comfort.**

Many of us were brought up with poor nutritional habits and consequently think – or most often *don't think* – that it's OK to eat rice and pasta every day. But believe me, there is nothing *fine* about *refined* food. Now there may be some cognitive dissonance kicking in with the few who may be thinking,

"I eat fine. I have cereal for breakfast, sushi for lunch and a frozen dinner. I'm not doing anything wrong."

And this is where you need to see that these choices are all poor choices because:

It's ALL PROCESSED FOOD

You have little to no idea how it was made or how many corners were cut to get you that food for cheap!

Now some people literally cannot even see food without desperate hunger kicking in. If this is you then this is what you'll need to get over to get healthy and fit. You don't always need to eat just because everyone else says that it's time. You need to begin to view food as just a way of replenishing your body with good clean fuel that allows it to run smoothly. Even if your body may currently resemble an SUV, start thinking of it more as a high performance, scorching hot sports car. Now if you owned a sexy sports car, would you use the cheapest gas in the tank? **Or would you treat it to the finest, cleanest, high-octane fuel?**

Yes, that's a no-brainer because you know you'd *always* give it the best so that it *gives you* the best performance. Well, it's the same for your body and it's the same for your food.

And *passive-aggressive eating – starving yourself all day in front of your co-workers only to binge at night –* won't ever work! Instead, you should re-channel that energy and devote your best effort to **eating yourself thin.** It's time to respect your hunger and eat as much delicious, healthy food as you want. Then, as your weight decreases, your stomach – and your appetite – will shrink which will lead directly to eating less.

There is also a bit of **FOMO** going on with shit food. FOMO is- *Fear Of Missing Out,* and you can see this in adverts for things like the rib sandwich at a certain fast food shop (gazillions served), or when it's that time of the year to eat (insert high-carb food here). How blatantly obvious is the misleading fast food marketing? What you are served is miles away from what the advert looks like. It is marketing based on legal bait and switch tactics.

Have you seen those commercials for people with heartburn who are encouraged to gulp down an antacid tablet/drug for relief?

Well, can you guess what's even better than an antacid drug?

Not eating a fucking chilli-and-cheese hot dog!

Let's not figure out ways to trick our body into eating a whole pizza... *let's just **not** eat it!* Instead, let's actually get a rush from turning down the French fries for a change.

The vast majority of the people I've interviewed shamefully expressed to me that a layer of fat on their body felt like a buffer between them and the world. It makes them feel safe and not as exposed even if they're embarrassed with themselves. What we need to do is break this connection between fat and *safe* and make you begin to feel comfortable with where you want to be.

When did you decide to be overweight? I've never gotten a clear answer on this question because no one ever "decided" to be fat... it just happened over time through woeful negligence. In many ways, I believe that being fat is like being homeless. If you became homeless overnight, you would spend all of your time trying to find a place to stay. If you are just realizing that you are fat, you should spend a lot of time figuring out a way to lose the weight. If you were dealt a bad hand by your parents, you have to move on from it and this plan is how you're going to get out of it. You're living in the most interesting era ever and you have this beautifully complex body that will take the best out of food and make it work for you. So why would you put anything foul in it? Why would you choose to be fat? Or poor? Or stupid? How can you **not** at least try to change the most viscerally constant and unsatisfying aspect of your life?

The one part of your life that you absolutely, indisputably can change!

Have you ever noticed that when friends overindulge on food, they always feel the need to explain why (i.e. *"It's Friday..."* or *"I'm bringing some back for my cubicle mate")?* It's because they're embarrassed and ashamed. This public anxiety leads to passive aggressive eating at home behind closed doors. We all see the results of this destructive behaviour and...*We need to stop this bullshit!*

People who are fit look at fat people eating candy bars as if they were smokers sucking down cancer. Sure you feel bad for them because they're caught in a trap and one of the most painful aspects of watching this slow suicide is that you can't openly talk to fat people (*or smokers*) about this without looking and sounding like a condescending prick (this is also why you write a book about it and have one of their friends give it to them as an anonymous gift). Just like a smoker, a fat person will defend their body type and blame others for asking them to change. Can you imagine how many billions are indirectly behind the campaigns for women to look natural, and be big and "proud" of their dangerously unhealthy size? There's no money in telling people to eat healthy, eat Paleo or to skip dessert.

I'm not making money off of it but, clearly, if I were a producer of sugary food, of course I'd make it my mission to cater to the Orca-sized. It would be my bread and peanut butter.

I'm going to make a generalization here, and I'm perfectly willing to cop shit for it. Just like every smoker wishes they could stop smoking, I know that every fat person wishes they could lose the weight and be fit. *They wish they could be in the position that you are about to find yourself –*

Becoming and being a person who is aware of exactly what you're eating and why.

Living a logical and easy path to lose weight and keep it off.

Doing it without surgery or unsustainable fad diets.

Eating shit is a confidence trick that most everyone falls for at some point. Even intelligent people fall for it until they find out they've been had and decide to make changes. No one makes healthy takeaway food. What you need to do is to *make your own healthy takeaway.*

So what is this undeniable draw to takeaway food that has cars lining up drive thrus? The simple answer is...

Convenience

We all know it's much more convenient to eat shit because:

It's readily available everywhere and

It's more profitable to create low-cost, high-caloric shit than healthier food.

Some foods that taste really good are the lowest version of barely edible food available. You think a hot dog at Coney Island or a cheesesteak in Philly is good food? It's the dregs. Fast food smells good because of all the chemicals pumped into them, which is why you're mindlessly in heaven when you walk into those places. It's the chemicals in the air tricking your brain into believing you're having a broiled 100% meat patty when it's really, *really* nothing like that.

When you go into a convenience store you should recognize how much shit there is to buy. There is usually *nothing* of any real nutritional value and *everything* is loaded with disgusting preservatives that will make it last for months on the shelf, just in case no one buys it.

It is now your duty to be conscious of what you're about to eat and then if it's not healthy...*simply don't eat it.*

It will take a few days to get over the sugar addiction but you can tame this craving with protein shakes. Eventually, the sugar addiction simply fades away. When that happens, you can pity the others caught in the sugar trap ordering pizza and diet soda (which is like taking a flame thrower to any hopes of getting in shape).

7

What Not To Eat

So let's talk about what **not** to eat.

Refined carbohydrates are the healthy-look killer. You don't want to eat any of these when you're trying to lose weight.

What are carbohydrates (carbs)?

Carbohydrates are molecules that consist of carbon, and hydrogen and oxygen atoms (hence their name). The healthy way of eating allows for carbs coming from vegetables and beans. They give you vitamins and help with the digestive process. Ideally you want them to come from Mother Earth and **not** from a factory. Factory-made carbs are called *refined carbohydrates*.

This means that *pasta, rice, bread*, and *cereal* are **bad, bad, bad, bad.** Drinks that have refined carbs are off the list, too. This means *beer, wine, soft drinks,* and *energy drinks* are **bad, bad, bad, bad.**

Are you ready to stop eating pasta, bread, cereal, and rice?

Sugar

Now what's the main ingredient I try to leave out of my healthy meals? *Sugar.*

Sugar is a type of carbohydrate. In its many forms, sugar triggers our frenemy insulin to be secreted by the pancreas.

When you have insulin in your blood stream, your body will look to use glucose from the ingested food before it uses stored fat.

Your body will always work on the path of least resistance. Sugar is easier to metabolize for energy than stored fat. Your body is hardwired to like sweet things because evolution has led us to believe that these foods contain a high amount of energy. Great when we are hunter gatherers, not so great when we can mass produce sugar.

So you may be unconsciously addicted to sugar but sugar is absolutely anathema to what we're trying to accomplish. If you aren't ready to give it up, you're not ready for this plan.

Fat is stored energy. Picture the fat on your body standing there in a line, waiting to be used next for a long walk or to climb stairs. Then right before it reaches the front of the line, sugar comes along and jumps in front so that the fat just sits there and makes you feel bad about it.

It's pretty simple: *If you have sugar in your regular meals or snacks, it will be a Sisyphean task to try to lose weight.*

So does this simply mean to cut out the candy bars and assorted crap?

What about those "socially acceptable sugars" as in steaming crois-sants or muffins in the morning?

The truth is that it's so much more than that.

Eventually you want to cut out all insulin triggers. Basically everything at a molecular level ending in *"ose"* is a sugar- *Glucose, sucrose, malt-ose, lactose, dextrose, fructose* and don't forget starch.

You may be reading that and thinking "Fructose"...*as in fruit?*

WTF Rudy?

Fruit always gets a dietary pass because people generally think about it as providing fiber and vitamins. It is still, *ultimately,* a form of sugar. It still spikes your insulin which switches off the burning of your stored fat. So am I saying to never eat fruit again?

Of course not.

I eat fruit when I want. What I *am* saying is that if you're trying to lose weight, fruit will only slow the process down. One of the crazier things that fructose can do is build up a resistance to *leptin*, which is the hormone that signals when you're full, or satisfied. So by eating more fruit you can artificially increase your appetite, which is actually *counterproductive* for anyone trying to lose weight.

And please pay attention:

A fruit smoothie is just a bunch of fruit blended together which puts even more fructose into your body than you can get from eating each fruit one at a time and eventually becoming full. Fruit juices and fruit smoothies are an unnecessary evil for the person trying to lose weight. You can get fiber from other sources and all of your vitamins from a multi-vitamin.

Fiber (which is actually a misnomer because many dietary fibers are *not* fibrous), in my most scientific of definitions, gets your bowels moving. I don't mean to burst your bubble on that, but it's just something you can't process. All fiber is made of carbohydrates that cannot be digested by the body's enzymes so it usually gets pretty far through you before being fermented by bacteria, or "gut flora." There are around *100 trillion* of these gut flora microorganisms in our intestines – *which is 10 times the amount of cells we actually have in our body* – and science still hasn't even been able to identify all of the gut flora species yet as many cannot be cultured. *Dietary Fiber* increases the weight and size of your stool which helps to decrease your chances of being constipated. It's generally considered to perform other functions like lower cholesterol levels and help to make you feel full, but we won't get into that. For the plan, the sources of fiber are in the beans and veggies that are in the meals. This is a good link regarding gut flora:

http://tinyurl.com/qx5movd

I shouldn't need to explain that high-fructose corn syrup is a huge part of our obesity problem, so all sugary drinks like **sports drinks, soda, alcohol,** and even all **flavoured waters** need to be put on hold when you're trying to lose weight. All of these are jam packed (ouch) with sugar, and if companies *could* put more sugar into food, they *would*, in order to lock you into your addiction. This is a great video explaining exactly how addictive it can be:

http://tinyurl.com/mje6zne

And what happens when sugary drink sales start slipping? They blame the consumer.

http://tinyurl.com/ogf45v6

Sugar is also a pro-inflammatory food.

Inflammation is needed in the body to protect itself when it's injured (i.e. the process of healing from a nick or cut) but when you have *chronic* inflammation it produces that internal "on fire" sensation related to conditions such as *heartburn, acid reflux, constipation* and conversely, *diarrhoea*. These are all signs that your body is not processing food correctly and, scientifically speaking...it's out of whack. Sugar is an inflammatory food, just like those containing *trans-fats, dairy products, MSG, flour, omega-6 oil, gluten* and it's also found in *alcohol*. As you get older it becomes increasingly difficult for your body to break these sugary substances down (I can't tell you how many of my friends and family have confided in me that they've been in serious pain internally and then discovered that they've become lactose intolerant or something similar). This breakdown in our digestive process is most likely because of the synthetic and man-made diet that our bodies are simply not evolved to process.

Perhaps you've heard this all before.

But I believe that what happens in our modern society is that we all tend to buy things that say they're *low in fat, sugar or carbs* and/or *high in fiber.* We trust that some corporation will look out for us with reliable science backing their protein bars, cereals, granolas, etc.

And so I'm here to tell you that these "low-fat", "reduced sugar", "high-fiber" products are all...*a bunch of bullshit.*

Like I said, anything that needs to tell you it's "good for you", *is not good for you*!

And because so many of us are brainwashed by these "healthy" labels and are convinced that we're eating a "healthy cereal" (another oxy-moron), of course some people think that maybe...*two helpings might be even "healthier" than one!*

And that is the entire purpose of all processed food – *It's modified to make you crave more of it.* They modify it so that you want more and make it easier for you to order the fries and soda to go with it. All processed foods give you a dopamine high that eventually bot-toms out while you're chemically brainwashed into feeling "full" and "satisfied", when in reality you've just dropped a dirty bomb inside of your body.

I don't, however, want you to quit sugar altogether but I do want you to **quit craving it.**

Craving is the real killer.

One can of soda contains about 8 teaspoons of sugar. For your body, all that sugar has the same effect as drinking a slow poison. If you have a proclivity to gain weight, then consider yourself *allergic to sugar* as long as you're trying to lose weight.

Am I asking you to give up *cakes, pastries, milk, fruit (yes, fruit),* and anything else containing sugar? Yes, I am. There will, however, always be a healthy amount of sugar in other foods that *are* allowed in the plan so we need never fear any shortage of the bad stuff.

Here are some scary numbers linking sugar with poor health and even death.

http://tinyurl.com/pmtcksh

Drinking Is Fun...But It's Not Helping

People often ask me questions about my work-out and diet "secrets".

Do you do Crossfit?

Lift weights?

Run?

Do you fast/cleanse/Paleo/gluten-free?

The good news is that my "secret" is:

1) *Consistency in my work-outs*
2) *Consistency in my eating habits*
3) *No more alcohol*

Of course, for many *that's also the bad news!*

I consciously gave up alcohol for a month to tweak my testosterone levels, and then after a month of looking and feeling increasingly fantastic, I kind of thought to myself,

"Why the hell have I been doing that each weekend for half of my life anyway?"

I felt like I'd woken up from a lazy slumber and I felt an enormous boost in my energy as well as an increasing drive to find my purpose in life. Maybe my mind was finally undoing the years of abuse that I'd put it under with dopamine addiction but the overall change was so positive and dramatic that I just kept going. In my case and yours, you can feel like you've been born again.

Now listen, my friend Tarus has told me (in reference to cigarettes),

"There's nothing worse than a reformed smoker..."

And to a great extent I agree with him but, take it from this "reformed" drinker, if you want to get fit fast and stay that way, *drinking doesn't help!*

Do you drink?

You can use this site to put your drinking into context.

http://tinyurl.com/qf4oywj

For a male, drinking a six-pack of Dutch beer is considered "binge drinking". Most men are only supposed to have 3-4 units of alcohol per day. This works out to 2 Dutch beers (no brand names please). Now think about it, can you ever *really* have only 2 beersies?

If you can, then you're a more disciplined drinker than I was because I usually had 6 to 8+ (emphasis on PLUS) on a Friday or Saturday night.

Now all alcohol has *7 calories per gram*, which is *significantly more than sugar* and other carbs which have only 4. So drinking is *literally* among the worst things you can do for weight loss, because it is so deceptively inconspicuous. At least when it comes to the bag of chips or gallon of ice cream, you know you're cheating. But with drinking, we "think" it just, "goes through me", or that "it's good for me", referring to red wine. Well, all alcohol is enormously high in calories, and consequently is even worse than eating because, considering our individual tolerance levels, it takes longer to get "full."

Picture a beer as being full of refined carbs and having as many calories as a mini-cheeseburger. Now think of eating 8 mini-cheeseburgers when you're out with your friends, then at the end of the night, throw in a kebab on your way home. Would that ever be a good thing? Granted, you may pass a great deal of the beer out and thus not retain all of the calories (*as we never own beer, we just rent it*) but it still seriously damages any weight loss or workout gains you're trying to achieve. It doesn't cause weight gain as much as it inhibits muscle growth and weight loss. In other words-*It keeps you fat.*

Am I saying that I'll never drink again? No. But it is all escapism. Your mind is tricked into trying to escape from itself each week. Once you drink, you've had a high and you bottom out looking for the next fix to get back there. It's the same with any recreational drugs or smoking. Once you can visualise this, and realise the grip it has on your mind, giving up drinking or smoking or anything that makes you escape (i.e. TV, and in our case overeating) is absolutely easy. Thinking clearer is so much better for your job, your relationship and the role model you project to kids.

So just know that one beer or a wine isn't going to ruin your physique, and if you can stop there, that's great. But just think, if you have a goal "weight", are you comfortable with making your goal "wait" just so that you look cool at a party? Your choice.

8

The Switch

Eating Healthy/Eating Clean

It may sound preachy and a bit like tough love, but if weight loss is the primary reason you're reading, I'm going to assume that other weight loss methods you've tried just didn't work and that you may need some strict guidelines set.

Well, you've come to the right place because it took me *years* to figure out that these are the best meals for not only losing weight but also keeping it off. You get to learn these hard-won lessons in just *minutes*! Lucky you.

Health writers tend to hide behind the line "individual results may vary..." but I'm going to state unequivocally that **this plan will work for anyone!** It's my Plan, and my book, so I feel confident making this statement. And like Kanye says –

"If you can do it better than me, then you do it."

Now can you identify yourself in one of these cycles?

You eat poorly → You have low energy → You find an excuse instead of working out → Your body and health continue to deteriorate

or

You eat healthy → You have a high energy level→ You attack your work-outs → You love the results and you love your body

The key is to *eat healthy first.* The rest will fall into place later.

For me, it's completely normal to eat healthy food, but it could be considered extreme for others. You could ease into this by lowering your calorie count each day, every week, but if you want to lose weight quickly, I'm giving you the meals that will kick your extra weight right in the ass! These meals work like gangbusters and *you can eat as many as you want* the whole time too. This is how you can **eat yourself thin** because one key thought I want you to keep in mind at all times is:

Fit people are never hungry because they can eat whenever they want!

In most self-improvement courses, the usual healthy lifestyle mix is:

A balanced diet combined with hitting the gym a few times a week.

This type of action is valid and can't hurt but, for my path, the gym part begins way after the eating. And I mean *way, way after*. Working out is of course beneficial, but healthy eating is the key to making a significant, lasting difference.

Also, there's simply no point in working out if you're still eating crap because you're only playing an ultimately self-defeating, and unhealthy, game. You will never get 6 *or* 8 pack abs – no matter how many "Ab Attack" classes you take – if you're still eating unhealthy food. To put things into further perspective, if you did a circuit training class and busted your butt to work off 500 calories, you would negate it and put those calories right back when you guzzle a sports drink. Now think about how much a poorly constructed lunch of crap puts back on after one of those classes. 3 times that amount? Perhaps 4 or more? The truth is that you will not lose the weight until you completely understand exactly what type of fuel you're putting into your awesome body machine.

And remember, I don't want you *to even think about working out until at least 3 months go by filled with healthy eating*. After those initial

3 months – *and after changing your eating habits for the better* – then you should start looking at your work-out options like going to the gym, or running, or basic home workouts. That's a later chapter, though, so let's focus on eating for now because this is where we get to have some fun!

Macronutrients

What is a macronutrient?

The prefix "macro" means large and nutrients are substances needed for growth, metabolism, and for other body functions. So "macros" are nutrients we need in large amounts in order to give us the bulk of energy to function properly. Of course our bodies require other additional nutrients which include vitamins but these nutrients are required in smaller quantities and are called *micronutrients*. While critical to our health, micronutrients *do not* provide us with energy or calories.

There are *3 major macronutrients* that the human body needs in order to function properly-

Carbohydrates

Protein

Fats

The amount of calories in each macronutrient varies, but it's pretty easy to remember this way:

Carbs and *Protein* provide *4 calories per gram*.

Fat provides *9 calories per gram*.

Now let's take a closer look at all three.

Carbohydrates (Carbs)

Carbohydrates primarily consist of sugar and starches and are our main source of fuel. All of the tissues and cells in our bodies can use glucose (from carbs) for energy. Given this nutritional reality, you cannot completely remove carbs from your diet as some fad dieting plans suggest because doing so would dramatically slow you down then leave you feeling weakened and sluggish. You *need* carbs, especially if you're going to eventually build muscle, but you should be eating healthy carbs only, as in *vegetables* and *beans*. If your primary goal is to lose weight then you want to stay away from all refined foods. The more a food has been *processed* the less work your body has to do to digest it so, consequently, processed foods are digested faster, allowing you to consume more calories while eating. If you consume these processed foods, you'll not only be hungry quicker (*because of the reduced time in digestion*) but you will also tend to eat more often throughout the day. Therefore,

Stay away from refined/processed foods and you'll feel full longer and not have to regret it later!

Simple *carbs* are those that can easily be metabolized, and these include *fruit, milk,* and *regular table sugar. Complex carbs* consist of larger molecules and require more time and energy from your body to metabolize. Complex carbs include *vegetables, beans* and *unrefined grains* (e.g. whole wheat or whole meal ones). For my body building readers, simple carbs will be needed later. For readers focused on weight loss, you want to stick with *complex carbs in small amounts,* but stay away from *grains and pasta* until you're happy with your results. If you want to keep a rough estimate of the percentage of carbs/fat/protein, go with 30%. Almost one- third of your meals should be carbs.

Fat (also known as Dietary Fat)

If you thought it sounds crazy that you *should be* eating carbs every day, get ready for this:

You have to not only eat fatty foods...you have to eat them every day!

We need *good fat* in our diets so that we can absorb fat soluble vitamins like vitamins *A, D, E* and *K*. Good fat can and will be used to keep inflammation down. But before we get into the types you should be eating, let's *discuss all of the types*.

There are *3 Main Fat Types:*

Trans-fats

Saturated fat

Unsaturated fat (which includes monounsaturated and polyunsaturated that are liquid at room temperature)

Trans-Fat

By far the most damaging type is **trans-fat**. This is a type of unsaturated fat, but made through a process called *partial hydrogenation.* This chemical process allows for oil to remain solid at room temperature which you can imagine is great for food manufacturers that want a longer shelf life for their products. Some restaurants also use this type of fat in their deep fryers so they don't (and won't) have to change the oil as often.

What makes trans-fat so toxic is that it raises the levels of *low-density lipoprotein LDL* (what is commonly referred to as the "bad cholesterol" that builds up in your arteries) and they simultaneously reduce the levels of the *high-density lipoprotein HDL* (considered as the "good cholesterol", the type that mops up excess cholesterol then returns it to your liver). To top off all the trans-fat bad news, current food labelling guidelines in the U.S. allow for an item to display *"0 grams of trans-fat"* even when that item contains up to 0.5 grams! This can quickly add up if you obliviously consume just a few *"trans-fat-free"* products.

The biggest offenders are:

Baked goods (cakes, ready-made icing, muffins, cookies and crackers made with shortening, which is partially hydrogenated vegetable oil)

Potato/corn/tortilla chips

Popcorn

Anything fried (French fries, doughnuts, fried chicken)

Margarine.

All those things may be considered tasty, but are absolutely the worst type of garbage to consume for anyone trying to lose weight. These are all horrible, body-killing, soul-destroying choices.

Saturated Fat

The next type of fat we'll discuss is **saturated fat**.

These mostly come from animal fat products such as:

Cream

Cheese

Butter

Meat

In addition, certain vegetables are high in saturated fat such as:

Coconut oil

Palm oil

Chocolate

Like trans-fats, these also raise your LDL levels, and they should be used sparingly (but definitely in place of trans-fats if you *have to choose* between the two). These fats are also solid at room temperature.

Unsaturated Fat

This brings us to **unsaturated fat**, which is the healthy or good fat that actually helps to lower your cholesterol levels.

Unsaturated fats are good fats primarily divided into:

Monounsaturated fat (MUFA)

Polyunsaturated fat (PUFA)

The difference between the two is a double bond in the fatty acid chain, but let me avoid putting you to sleep by going down that road. Suffice to say that *both* of these types of unsaturated fat are generally *liquid* at room temperature.

Examples of monounsaturated fats are:

Nuts

High fat fruits like *olives* and *avocados*

Polyunsaturated fats can be found in:

Flaxseeds

Walnuts

Canola and olive oil

Sunflower and sesame seeds

Sardines and salmon

Fish oil

Soybeans

Tofu

Unsalted peanuts and peanut butter

And this is where **Essential Fatty Acids** (EFA's) come into play.

These are fats that are required by our own bodies for biological processes but cannot be synthesized or produced within our bodies. If we don't get these fatty acids into our system, we develop deficiencies and run the risk of becoming ill.

There are 2 EFA's:

Omega-3 fatty acid (commonly called alpha-linoleic acid)

Omega-6 fatty acid (commonly called linoleic acid)

I wrote that fat *can help* with inflammation, and that is exactly what omega-3 fatty acid does. It is very beneficial for those with chronic inflammation, examples being *ulcers, arthritis, colitis and sinusitis*. Basically, anything that has an "itis" in the word should also come with a daily dose of fish oil to counteract it. I myself take 1 capsule of fish oil with every meal (1.5 grams each). If you are battling any chronic inflammation I highly recommend fish oil as an effective daily remedy.

If you want to maintain a rough estimate of the percentage of fat/protein/carbs, go with 30%. Almost *one-third of your meals* should be unsaturated fat.

Protein

This brings us to our very good friend, Protein, who you will need to be even closer to. Proteins are the building blocks of our life. They are nutrients essential for the human body and absolutely crucial in building other proteins, enzymes and hormones that are vital for normal functioning. Protein makes up our skin, hair, nails, bones and so much more. For this nutrient, I want you to say these words OUT LOUD:

"PROTEIN WILL NEVER MAKE ME FAT!"

Say it loud, say it proud. Protein *cannot make you fat* as your body simply doesn't work that way. Protein is made up of amino acids and there are about 500 known aminos in existence. Out of those 500, the human body needs certain aminos on a daily basis in order to continue functioning. The nonessential ones are ones that our bodies can make on our own. The essential ones are ones that need to be in our daily food. They are listed here:

Essential	Nonessential
Histidine	Alanine
Isoleucine	Arginine
Leucine	Aspartic acid
Lysine	Cysteine
Methionine	Glutamic acid
Phenylalanine	Glutamine
Threonine	Glycine
Tryptophan	Proline
Valine	Serine
	Tyrosine
	Asparagine
	Selenocysteine

Wouldn't life be so much easier if there were simply foods that contained all of these amino acids? Well guess what, there are: eggs, legumes, soy and whey.

Eggs are the "Ragu" of food choices...*It's in there!*

There's a convenient method of evaluating protein adopted by the U.S.F.D.A. and it can be found here:

http://tinyurl.com/p7anh5a

It ranks protein sources with *egg whites, soy protein, whey and casein* coming out on top, followed then by *beef*. This eating plan we're working on loves all of these sources. Eggs, of course, go great with almost any breakfast, and the other three proteins are readily available in most protein shakes.

Protein is the most satiating, satisfying type of nutrient and has the direct potential to keep you feeling full far longer than either carbohydrates or fats.

If you want to keep a rough estimate of the percentage of protein/carbs/fat, go with 40%. Almost *half of your meals* should be protein. Counting macronutrients is a very simple way to look at meals. You will always count macros once you understand them. Get your macros right and weight loss will be a breeze.

Now let's get into what *we should be eating*!

9

What's Really Good for Our Bodies?

Let's make one point perfectly clear:

To lose weight, you DO NOT want to – nor have to – starve yourself!

Starving yourself is not only counterproductive but doomed to fail. When deprived of proper nutrition, the body goes into *starvation mode.* In starvation mode, the body actually *holds onto the fat* that you're starving yourself to lose. What you want to do is to drop the weight by eating healthy food – and more of it than ever before. By eating food that's *higher in protein and lower in fat and carbs*, you will feel satiated for longer periods. Since protein has less than half the calories of fat, *you will be able to effectively lose weight by eating more.*

So what you have in your fridge and pantry is the key to it all because your eating is going to dictate how your body looks in the next 3 months...and then for the rest of your life!

To put it simply, from now on, you want to eat *Single Ingredient Foods.* This Plan can perhaps be best understood as a unique variation of the popular *Paleo diet* (look it up if you haven't heard about it yet) with elements of the Zone diet included. That being said, my Plan is healthier because it's not as extreme as either version and it's more easily followed because it doesn't force you to compulsively obsess over constant measuring and stressing about what exactly is or isn't *Paleo.*

Here is a list of the tasty, delicious and nutritious foods that you can eat daily in your First 3 Months:

Eggs

Eye fillet steak (beef tenderloin in the States)

Fresh chicken breasts

Fish

Canned beans (look for high-protein varieties)

Vegetables (frozen is fine, the bags with veggie mixes work great)

Spinach (frozen is fine as well)

Garlic (buy it crushed so you don't need to clean a press)

Hot sauce and mustard (luxury taste kick)

All of these basics should be easily available almost everywhere and none of them should strain your budget any more than takeaway food would.

Now if, for any reason, you can't find these exact basics...relax. *It's the principle that matters.* As long as you continue to eat strictly high-protein/low-sugar meals, you'll be fine.

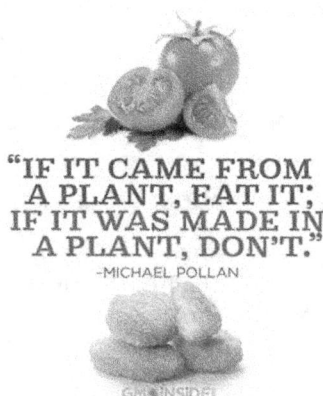

"IF IT CAME FROM A PLANT, EAT IT; IF IT WAS MADE IN A PLANT, DON'T."
-MICHAEL POLLAN

GMO INSIDE
Coalition Powered by Green America

You may have noticed that these foods are basically a derivative of the aforementioned *Paleo diet.* It's a great set of ideas, but Paleo hardliners tend to get stuck on the idea of only being allowed to eat foods that were around prior to the Agricultural Revolution. This is *paralysis by analysis.* We want to avoid this counterproductive activity and keep moving forward! If you can find fresh, unprocessed food, it doesn't matter if it was around during caveman times. So don't stress out trying to *keep up with the Paleo dogma.* Just eat fresh. Just eat unprocessed.

As far as drinking goes, this is often the most insidiously subtle way that most of us unknowingly turn off the fat burning switch and gain weight. So I'm going to say it again:

All flavoured drinks have sugar in them!

The sugar is what gives it that "flavour". So as harmless as it may seem to gulp a *smart water, sports drink, fruit juice or soda,* they all turn off your fat burning switch.

Take the worst of these, the soda. When you count the calories on a can or bottle of soda and compare it to the same amount of calories in vegetables, you'll clearly see that it's frightening how much more can be packed into something we normally think of as simply a "drink".

In these first 3 months you should be drinking:

Water

Water

And

Only water

This means with *ALL of your meals.*

Sound difficult, disappointing, or just plain too boring for you? Well, I can 100% guarantee you that there weren't any cavemen slugging down soft drinks way back when. And I'd personally much rather drink water with my meals for *3 short months* than be forced to hide like a fugitive every time I passed a mirror *for the rest of my life!* Water accelerates weight loss so try to get your water consumption up to 2-3 litres a day. Yeah, that much.

Vitamins

The biggest, most consistent gripe about the Paleo diet is that it simply does not provide all the necessary vitamins and nutrients we all require to be healthy. I will not try to argue this.

It's well known that deficiencies in common vitamins such as A, B12, C, and D can lead to some pretty nasty disorders such as blindness, anaemia, scurvy, and rickets. Our bodies can synthesize some vitamins but as humans continue to evolve, this ability to synthesize tends to decrease because so many vitamins are in dietary abundance. No need to waste energy making your own when there's a plentiful source just inside the refrigerator door.

Remember the *essential fatty acids* from the last chapter? The ones we need each day but can't make ourselves? Well allow me to introduce you to their close cousin: *the essential nutrient*. Our body requires these nutrients (including vitamins) every day.

What I do each day to ensure that I get all the essential nutrients is take a multi-vitamin (or "multi"). That covers everything I require. I prefer an Optimum Nutrition variety called "Opti-Men". For women, there is the "Opti-Women" (the difference being smaller portions of vitamins yet higher in iron). Multis can and do provide a reliable, nutritional stopgap and back-up for any vitamins you might be lacking.

There's a theory regarding cravings common to pregnant women and how these cravings are simply the body calling out for the nutrients that it's temporarily lacking in sufficient numbers (think ice cream and pickles). I believe it's the same for everyone else: Your body knows what it needs and can compel you to eat certain things if there's a deficit in your diet. If you take a multi, you'll cover yourself nutritionally and conveniently avoid eating anything detrimental simply because your body has a temporary craving. Finding it hard to stay awake? This could be a lack of vitamin B12 in your diet. Do you have good sources of cobalamin in your food? Ha. Multis will help to fight this fatigue.

Think of them as *nutritional insurance* for any type of nutritional deficit you may encounter. They, along with fish oil, should become a staple in your everyday life.

Now hear this!

If you read this book and still can't/don't/won't work-out...that's fine.

If you can't/don't/won't cook for yourself and eat yourself thin...that's fine too.

If you can't/don't/won't take fish oil every day...fine.

But please start taking a multi every day. Whether it's a supermarket brand or the Optimum Nutrition products, multis are key to controlling your body. If baby steps are your thing, *please make that first step a daily multi.*

Check this site to see if your favourite supplements are the real deal:

http://tinyurl.com/p5s2uft

10

"Yes, I Eat Cow. I Am Not Proud"

The title for this very brief chapter comes to us thanks to the late, great Kurt Cobain and yes...

I do eat cow. I eat animals.

But before you run off to burn this book in your vegan BBQ's, allow me to explain. I don't really like to think about how meat ends up in my supermarket but I am also *not* a proponent for the inhumane treatment of animals. In the interest of complete transparency, I don't really believe that *free range* farming is doing animals any better than the standard type of farming. The ideals of free range farming should be applauded but the practice still leaves a lot to be desired. If there were a way to harvest chicken or steak humanely, I'd be all for that.

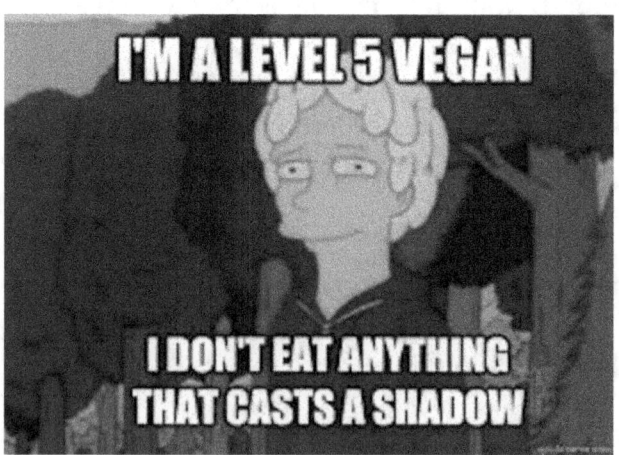

Further, I believe (and hope) that in 50 years, most of us will look back at our meat-processing industry and think about how barbaric it was to kill animals for protein when we could have manufactured it. Animal agriculture could be worse for our planet than cars even. In point of fact, if there were an efficient method for getting all the macronutrients out of other food options without killing any animals, I would be all over that in a heartbeat. But please don't tweet me about how chick-peas, legumes or quinoa will provide the same nutrients as meat. Yes, soy is a great protein provider but I just don't see myself eating tofu long term and I wouldn't ask anyone else to do it either. I also don't believe in the theory of non-violence as a reason to give up a diet. Your body is constantly killing bacteria inside of it, so you are already a killing machine. It is part of nature. Inhumanely doing it is morally wrong though. I don't know if you'd consider my ennui towards eating meat to be on par with human rights violations of the past and present and I'm sure my laissez-faire attitude bothers a few veggie warriors, but I realize I can't please everyone. There is an old Russian saying that states, *"If you eat fat, you become fat and if you eat meat you become meat..."*

Well...*I know which one I prefer to be.*

11

Mistakes we all Make
(but won't anymore)

Before we dive into food prep, I want to warn you about these 3 giant blindsides that can and *will* take your eyes off the prize. The first are those pesky things called "people."

Those Damn Other People

In one of my favorite episodes of "Seinfeld", Elaine brings up the subject of hating *"people"*, to which Jerry adamantly replies, *"Yeah, they're the worst."*

People can really take the wind out of your sails when you choose to listen to any "expert" who thinks they have all the "answers" when it comes to nutrition and fitness without any visible empirical evidence to back up their claims; kind of like a fat coach, a skinny chef or a single matchmaker. For example, some "experts" will tell you that sweetener is bad for you, even though you're choosing it over sugar. They'll tell you that using fluoride in your toothpaste is a government conspiracy when you only need to research *Antigo, Wisconsin*, or the Scottish towns of *Wick and Stranraer* to find real facts. If you took everyone's advice at the same time, you'd think that the very best carbon footprint you can leave is killing yourself.

Look...It's much easier to grab attention when you say or write something sensationalist, alarming or strictly for shock value. But what we really need to do is simply use common sense when we're considering our life options. You know what I mean?

If there is one thing true in literature, it is the sentence "Don't believe everything you read." Do I know everything? Of course not. I have an open mind though, and I'm always open to improvements and tweaks. If you don't implicitly trust what I'm writing, then good for you! You're on the right track but look a topic up first before you dismiss any information. Do some research and/or find your own happy way of doing it but don't just go with the flow or buy some crappy ab contraption off the TV because the model hawking it in the commercial was ripped.

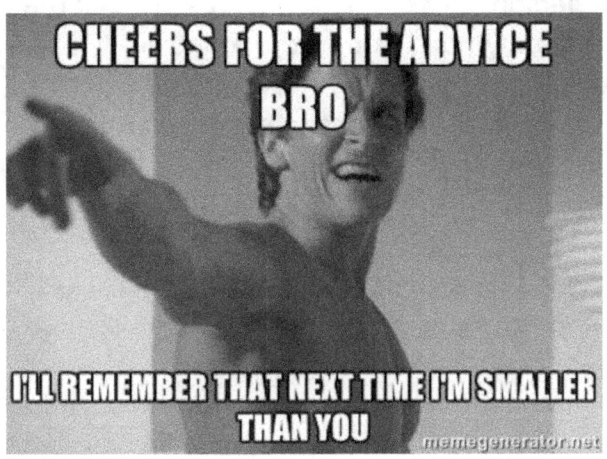

In my short time on Earth, the fittest people I've met are almost always humble and reserved about how and why they take care of their bodies. If you ask them for advice, of course they'll happily share but they're usually not *in your face* about any programs or plans and usually have no "health" axes to grind. The people who do spend their time proselytizing – *much like those eager to discuss their wealth or success* – are usually the ones who are the most insecure about what they do or where they fit in and the ones whose unsolicited advice is worth the least.

I Deserve...

This is one of the most toxic rationalizations that can really derail your progress moving forward. And I mean this in the most regressive terms. Think of those convenient occasions that will constantly crop up in which we give ourselves permission to fail by stroking our own egos with:

"I deserve (insert unhealthy food here) now because I've been good all day."

This is called *moral licensing*. And don't get me wrong, we've all seen or done this before. The most ridiculous example is when someone orders a diet soda to offset ordering that disgusting fast food burger. If you're that person, please realize that it's just a pathetic nutritional shell game that only hurts you in the long run. If you ever begin to feel that you've *lost some weight* so you're now entitled to *eat some shit* because...wait for it...**you deserve it**, then you're flying in the face of all the progress you painstakingly made and you're about to *crash and burn.*

We all tend to do this to justify any number of failings like alcoholism, racism, sexism or extremism. It all starts with those tired tropes:

"I deserve to have a drink because I haven't had one all week..."

"I deserve to have a cigarette when I drink because I don't when I'm not drinking..."

"I deserve to be racist in this one conversation because I've been so non-racist leading up to this..."

"I have all types of friends, so I deserve to be able to post this hurtful and mean-spirited thing on social media..."

"I deserve to have this minor indiscretion because I leave less of a carbon footprint than others..."

Those two words can be your downfall.

The Five Point Swing

I find that one of the most effective ways to realistically examine the sustained *action* of cutting weight is to understand that **you are actually losing weight every time you say NO to shit food!**

Think of it this way: In basketball, *a single play* can often be the difference between scoring *2* and the other team scoring *3*. When we examine that single play we can easily understand that it creates, in reality, a 5 point overall difference in the outcome of the whole game. Well... *It's the same for food!* When you say NO to shit food, you not only avoid the excess weight it directly causes, you also avoid having to lose that excess weight you would've otherwise packed on. In a very real way, you're actually *making a 5 point difference every time you say NO!*

A penny saved is definitely a penny earned in this sense. So think about that one play when you're cutting weight and take that lesson with you everywhere you go.

As just one example that occurs to me frequently, I often get the feeling that certain fatties shower me with pity whenever I choose to bring my own home-made protein lunch to any and every company sponsored buffet (provided gratis of course). Yes, it's much easier to eat a free trash-food meal than it is to eat a healthy meal you paid for yourself, but why would you want to willingly introduce warmed-over foulness from last week's freezer into your system and gratuitously sacrifice your health just to save a few bucks? Of course we can kid ourselves into believing that this single cheat/treat chow down would be an awesome break after a week of Spartan living, but if you want to get healthy and stay healthy then push it out to next week...and then the week...and then the next...until, one day, you're in front of the mirror, naked and happy at last and for the future!

I hope that my continued use of this naked metaphor doesn't get me sent selfies of naked people.

12

Your Kitchen is Your Kingdom

I'll start this chapter by repeating myself.

The key to eating healthy is to be in control of what you put into your body. The best way to do this is to cook your own food at home.

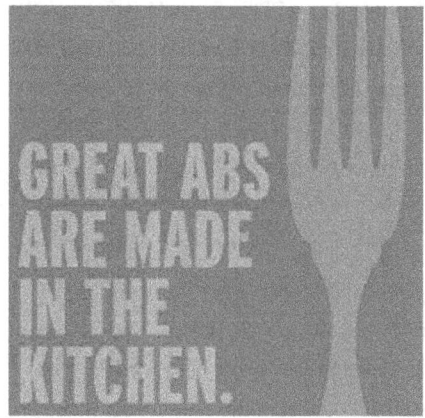

Cooking, much like working out, is not only the best, healthiest option for your body, it's also a great escape from the madness of life. When I need a break from my job during the day, *I work-out*. When I need a break from my home life, *I cook*. I've found that the best way to do this is to make your kitchen one of your favourite rooms in your humble abode.

Before I started eating healthy, I saw the kitchen as a bit of a no-man's land or a male no-fly zone. I had girlfriends who'd cook, but I always fell back on my duties as the trusty dish washer rather than get in there and wrestle the beast. Sure, I picked up a thing here or there, but ultimately I was of the mind-set that if I made a mess in there – *which I was sure I would* – then I'd also have to clean the mess...*so why not just get takeaway?*

Well, letting go of this irresponsible mind-set is another key to the program. Because from this point forward, you're going to have to embrace your kitchen and learn how to use all of the tools it contains. So let's get started with the very basics.

I'm going to recklessly assume you have a stovetop in your kitchen, with plates, bowls and utensils of some kind along with at least 1 clean kitchen towel. If you don't have these things, put this book down and go get them RIGHT NOW!

You also need to acquire these items (all of which can be sourced at any dollar shop):

1 pan (if you can afford a good one, I highly suggest Tefal non-stick)

3-5 small plastic containers with locking lids (1 litre or 32 oz. rectangles that can easily hold an entire meal)

1-2 large plastic containers with locking lids (2 litre or 68 oz. rectangles that can fit in your microwave)

1 pot

1 set of tongs

1 chopping board

1 egg whisker

1 roll of clingy plastic wrap

1 can of olive oil spray (to keep food from sticking or burning)

Simple enough?

If you have a microwave, that's a bonus. If not, use the pot to do fresh beans and the other pan for fresh veggies.

Once you've bought these items, it's good to understand your kitchen because you'll need to become *one* with it. It's another key to your success. So have a look at your stovetop. Is it gas or electric? How many ranges does it have? Even if you only have two, that's fine for our purposes but you will need to take the time and master the heat settings on your stovetop. I'm going to assume that your stovetop works so while you're getting familiar with it, why not give it a thorough clean down. Do you still have gunk all over from ages ago?

Put your OCD hat on and give it a good clean with some disinfectant and paper towels and don't spare the elbow grease. In fact, why not take this opportunity to get ahead of the game and use a few hours to clean your entire kitchen?

Here's an excellent piece of simple kitchen cleaning advice that you can apply to so many other areas of life:

Throw out the rubbish that you never use and don't need!

You need to make your kitchen your temple. Your temple should never be filled with trash so throw it out with extreme prejudice. Your kitchen needs to be an inviting place because soon it will become your portal to happiness.

And while we're throwing things out, do you happen to be holding onto a pantry or fridge stash of trashy treats?

Keeping trashy treats in your house is just begging for trouble. Don't let the money you spent on those treats keep you from your weight loss goals. Ask yourself:

How much would you spend to lose a few pounds?

Right...that's what I thought. So just chuck them out. Alternatively, you could give them away to your nearest hateful neighbour and hope he'll eat them all. That's a bit mean, isn't it? Whatever you do with that garbage, do it now. Don't wait.

If you're still trying to convince yourself that you're the thrifty type who eats everything just to save the money, you're not only kidding yourself but you're hurting yourself as well and making the whole process that much harder. Think about that when you bite into a cupcake or some chocolate chip cookie dough. It's going to take longer to get better so just

THROW IT AWAY NOW!

Lovely.

Getting back to the dishes, for those of you who don't yet know how to cook, these tools will be a good starter for you to get into the game. Your partner (or potential partner) will undoubtedly love this new skill of yours. So this is a skill that gives you exponential benefits in so many areas of your life.

Now let's make some delicious meals!

13

How to Cook Meals and Love it

Breakfast

Breakfast is almost always my favourite meal of the day. I always make it at the same time every day and it's become one of my most treasured rituals: daily prep, cook, eat, clean up, and launch my day. Perfect!

For those of you who don't bother yourself with breakfast (too busy, too lazy, too unprepared), this alone could be one big reason you're reading this book. When you skip meals, you get fatter over time because you'll always end up by overcompensating at other times in your day. When you skip breakfast, you'll absolutely accelerate your fat storage because eating bigger meals later on will be needed to keep your blood sugar levels elevated.

In fact, in the beginning I would go so far as to say that you can *and should* look at breakfast as your only pig-out meal of the day. You should eat as much as you want of the foods I'm suggesting because your body will burn it off much more efficiently than either a big lunch or late dinner. This is what we can safely call common sense. When you load up on protein in the morning it sets you up for the day. It's the opposite reaction when you have a low- or no-protein breakfast because the only thing you're setting yourself up for are constant cravings for more and more.

As to what you should eat for breakfast, I'll let you in on a little secret: *EGGS* are the miracle centrepiece of it all.

If you aren't eating eggs for breakfast yet, then my friend, you're in luck because this is one of the best food switches you'll make. Eggs are indeed a miracle food because they're pretty much all upside, with little to no downside. Almost any other breakfast food you can mention (pancakes, cereals, oatmeal, etc.) is strictly the opposite.

This is a great site on the benefits of eggs:

http://tinyurl.com/ocrmmqk

I myself tend to vacillate between *scrambled eggs, fried eggs* and *omelettes* depending on my mood. I usually cook with both eggs and additional *egg whites*.

I could inflict my personal egg recipes on you but for the purpose of convenience I'll just provide you with superb recipes from top notch chefs to get you on your way.

This site, Food52, is great.

http://tinyurl.com/qdvm3fm

If I had to choose only one of those as my last meal, I lean towards *The Classic Method*.

Here's a great French omelette.

http://tinyurl.com/pvhv8ub

Here's a great one for poached scrambled eggs.

http://tinyurl.com/pg5dwvv

Here is the macronutrient breakdown of my usual breakfast of eggs over easy/scrambled on bread:

4 Eggs

Protein: 24 g   Carbs: 2 g   Fat: 20 g

3 Egg Whites (roughly how much I pour from the pouch)

Protein: 9 g   Carbs: 0 g   Fat: 0g

Whole Grain Bread (totally optional)

Protein: 10 g   Carbs: 46 g   Fat: 4 g

Totals:

Protein: 43 g   Carbs: 48 g   Fat: 24 g

Just to reiterate, egg whites are basically all protein with no carbs or fat. In my diet plan, they're a magical wonder food that are basically all benefit. I used to think that *egg whites* meant that I had to separate the yolks from the whites but many supermarkets now sell pre-separated egg whites in a pouch.

Now let's compare this to the average fast food meal.

Bacon, Egg and Cheese Biscuit

Protein: 19 g   Carbs: 38 g   Fat: 26 g

And please keep in mind that this is for only one tiny sandwich that personally never satisfied me so I rarely ever stopped at just one. So when we take this not-so-unusual behaviour into account, we can see that one single tiny sandwich will leave you hungry for much more, and yet still overload you with carbs and fat, especially in comparison to a large, satisfying meal of eggs.

Now you can only imagine what the addition of the requisite orange juice & hash browns do to these levels. Cost and convenience can only go so far. If you're serious about cutting weight then you simply cannot afford to leave it in the hands of fast food franchises.

Eggs are much healthier and much more nutritionally satisfying than cereal or oatmeal. They're light years better than having nothing at all in the morning because eating nothing for breakfast is abusing your body. Your body is already in a state of ketosis from the previous night's sleep and it needs energy to get you moving.

Once you start eating a healthy breakfast, you'll get to a point where you'll ask yourself why you would pay big money for someone to cook your eggs for you. It just doesn't make sense when you learn how to do it yourself. I basically have the same equipment at home as a restaurant – a pan and a spatula – so I don't see the point in paying through the nose for some bloody eggs. Basic accounting and common sense informs me that it costs around $5 for smoked salmon and eggs. Yet because they add some tired parsley and a half-hearted smile at the café they wanna charge me $25? FOH!

That's breakfast.

Lunch & Dinner

Now that you've got a handle on eggs, let's move on to the meals that, along with breakfast, will allow you to lose all the excess weight you want to lose. And the best part about these meals you're going to prepare for yourself is that *you can eat as much of them as you like and still lose the weight!*

Here are my recommended meals to enjoy (this is subjective so if you can make other combinations with the food listed, feel free). If any of this is too hard to understand, it is essentially making a chicken lunch with beans and veggies, or a steak dinner with beans and veggies. Just make sure that you have high protein in EVERY meal. Substitute the chicken and steak for fish if you feel daring after a while.

Chicken Lunches (cook 3 lunches at a time, one time on Sunday night, and then Wed night)

3 fresh chicken breasts (which amounts to approximately 516 grams or 18 ounces)

With a good sharp knife, cut these into pieces about the size of a pinkie each.

Put the pan on the stove, spray with oil, and turn the heat to medium.

When the pan feels hot with your hand just over it, add the chicken, spacing it so that no one piece is on top of another.

Add in your favorite spices. I can't stress this enough. Chicken without spices is uber boring.

Cook for 4-5 minutes, making sure to move them every 30 seconds so that they don't stick to the pan.

Turn them all over and cook until done. Make sure to move any larger portions towards the middle of the pan as you go so that they cook through.

Check to see if they're done by slicing a bigger piece into two. Make sure the middles are cooked through.

When they're all cooked, turn the heat off, apportion the meat out to your containers or plate and *clean up!*

Steak Dinner - Eye fillet (called tenderloin in the US)

Take an eye fillet steak (135 grams or four ounces) out of your fridge and let it get to room temperature as you heat the pan up.

Put the pan on the stove, spray it with oil (heavily in the middle), and turn the heat to medium.

When the pan feels very hot with your hand over it, add the steak to the middle. Move it around a few times in the beginning as steak can stick very easily.

Let the steak cook for 4-5 minutes on one side, making sure to move it around every 30 seconds so that it doesn't stick.

Turn it over to the other side then cook it until done, making sure to move the steak so it doesn't stick.

Let the steak cook until you see the juices start to form on the top of the steak. This is *medium rare* (cook less or more depending on your taste). Now take it off and let it cool for a few minutes.

Turn the heat off and *clean up!*

Pork Tenderloin – *Same as steak*

Salmon or Tuna – *Same as steak*

Both *lunch and dinner* revolve around heating up frozen veggies.

1 large rectangle container (2-liter size)

1/2 bag of mixed frozen veggies (700 grams or roughly 32 ounces)

2 fist sized amounts of frozen spinach

Chopped garlic

1 can of beans (425 grams or 15 ounces). Black beans and butter beans are the highest in protein at my supermarket.

Add frozen vegetables and spinach to the 2L sized container (loosely put the lid on it to allow steam to get out) and place in microwave for 6 minutes on high.

Set the 3 containers open in front of their lids.

Open the can of beans and apportion them out evenly to the 3 containers.

Put 1 spoonful of chopped garlic in each container

If you have a minute or two to spare while you're waiting, start cleaning up and discarding wrappers and other items (this will make clean-up easier afterward).

When 6 minutes is up, check on the veggies. If they need another 2-3 minutes, spread them around and restart (usually my spinach balls need to be pressed with a fork and moved around a bit).

When your chicken is done (previous), apportion the chicken and veggies out to each of the containers evenly.

Put the lids on the containers, let them cool down then place in the fridge for your lunches.

Bring your lunch to work the next day and store in fridge. At lunchtime, heat it for 3 minutes on high in your work microwave and enjoy with a glass or two of water.

Voila. Job done.

Now here are the macronutrient breakdowns of these meals:

Chicken (172 grams)

Protein: 64 g   Carbs: 0 g   Fat: 24 g

Beans

Protein: 7 g   Carbs: 24 g   Fat: 1 g

Veggies

Protein: 7.5 g   Carbs: 7.5 g   Fat: 0 g

Totals:

Protein: 78.5 g   Carbs: 31.5 g   Fat: 25 g

Eye fillet/Beef tenderloin (1 steak at approximately 135 grams)

Protein: 38 g   Carbs: 0 g   Fat: 30 g

Beans

Protein: 7 g   Carbs: 24 g   Fat: 1 g

Veggies

Protein: 7.5 g   Carbs: 7.5 g   Fat: 0 g

Totals:

Protein: 52.5 g   Carbs: 31.5 g   Fat: 31 g

Salmon or Tuna (172 grams)

Protein: 39 g   Carbs: 0 g   Fat: 22 g

Beans

Protein: 7 g   Carbs: 24 g   Fat: 1 g

Veggies

Protein: 7.5 g   Carbs: 7.5 g   Fat: 0 g

Totals:

Protein: 54.5 g   Carbs: 31.5 g   Fat: 23 g

Pork (135 grams)

Protein: 42 g   Carbs: 0 g   Fat: 23 g

Beans

Protein: 7 g   Carbs: 24 g   Fat: 1 g

Veggies

Protein: 7.5 g   Carbs: 7.5 g   Fat: 0 g

Totals:

Protein: 56.5 g   Carbs: 31.5 g   Fat: 24 g

As you can see, quality meat (do not substitute any of these with inferior products like sausages or ground meat) is generally high in protein and fat and has zero carbohydrates. If you get your carbohydrate quota from veggies, you my friend, will be skinny in no time.

Now let's compare this to the average of a fast food meal.

Fast Food Burger with Toppings

Protein: 24 g   Carbs: 47 g (*yikes*)   Fat: 27 g

Large French Fries

Protein: 6 g   Carbs: 67 g (*yikes*)   Fat: 24 g

Large Cola

Protein: 0 g   Carbs: 76 g (*yikes*)   Fat: 0 g
(I defy anyone to find a soda that's significantly different.)

Totals:

Protein: 30 g   Carbs: 190 g   Fat: 51 g

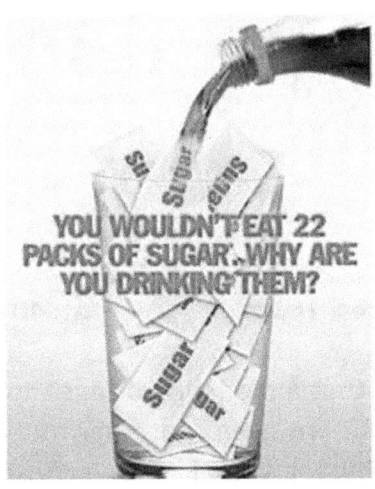

I almost started tearing up when I started adding up those numbers. This is just horrible abuse to your body in every way. With over 1200 calories in this fast food "meal", it should easily cover more than half of all your meals for the day...but of course it doesn't. Here's an interesting look at the standard restaurant meal and how it drastically explodes your caloric needs.

http://tinyurl.com/prcgta2

Perhaps you're thinking that chicken is the healthier choice at a fast food filling station?

Let's compare our chicken to the average of a fast food chicken "meal".

Grilled Chicken Burger

Protein: 14 g   Carbs: 40 g (*yikes*)   Fat: 16 g

Large French Fries

Protein: 6 g   Carbs: 67 g (*yikes*)   Fat: 24 g

Large Cola

Protein: 0 g   Carbs: 76 g (*yikes*)   Fat: 0 g
(There's those 76 g of sugar again!)

Totals:

Protein: 20 g   Carbs: 183 g   Fat: 40 g

You may be thinking that a diet soda brings the carb numbers down significantly, but these are even more harmful to your body. Again, not trying to be alarmist, just making you conscious of exactly what you're doing when you drink this poison. Check these sites for more details.

http://tinyurl.com/kqr29gu

http://tinyurl.com/nfz3a8c

How about a sandwich shop stop and 1 drinking water?

6-inch Chicken Strip sandwich

Protein: 22 g   Carbs: 37 g   Fat: 4 g

Non-White Bread

Protein: 8 g   Carbs: 30 g   Fat: 3 g

Totals:

Protein: 30 g   Carbs: 67 g   Fat: 7 g

And that's with **no toppings or dressing**! Now tell me (and more importantly, tell yourself), do you *really only order a single 6-inch* when you hit the sandwich shop? Well, if not then **double those numbers for the 12-inch!** I'm running out of yikes…

How about sushi and 1 drinking water?

Tuna Roll (6 pcs)

Protein: 24 g   Carbs: 27 g   Fat: 2 g

Salmon and Avocado Roll (6 pcs)

Protein: 13 g   Carbs: 42 g   Fat: 9 g

And this is with *no soy sauce or wasabi.*

Now do you normally stop at 6 pieces? 12? Well add them together if you normally eat 12 like I used to do. On their own, and at 6 pieces only, sushi is the best of the worst, but when you consider the molecular level of how the refined white rice will spike your insulin and the sodium from the soy sauce will make you retain water, these are really not a healthy alternative but more like the lesser of two evils.

The reason why I threw these comparisons into our mix is because these are typically some of the normal choices for the average 9-5er. Yet we have to understand *that all of these* are unhealthy options and anything outside of them, *as in Indian and Chinese food*, are really, really detrimental to any progress you're going to make.

Let me list out the foods that I think are good for your weight loss and why:

1. Eggs – the wonder food. Should be eaten every day as per the prior chapter.
2. Chicken – Has fat, but a good lean protein. Stick with chicken breasts.
3. Steak – All depends on the cut, but high in fat and protein. Stick with choice cuts like eye fillet, bottom round, top sirloin. Stay away from chuck and ground round.
4. Turkey – Another lean meat. Best to get it off the bone and not processed with god knows what.
5. Fish – Cod, haddock, salmon, tuna, and trout being the best.
6. Venison – Very high in protein. Great way to relieve the monotony of steak, fish and chicken all the time.
7. Kangaroo – much easier to find by my Aussie mates. Very high in protein.
8. Kudu, Oryx – much easier to find by my Saffa mates. Very high in protein. Oryx is the tastiest meat I've ever eaten in my life.
9. Most Vegetables – I use frozen ones myself and go heavy on spinach, broccoli, carrots, green beans, etc.

10. Nuts – Almonds, cashews. Stay away from blanched or honey roasted ones.

What to definitely NOT eat when you are trying to lose weight:

1. Anything with sugar in it – too many to list
2. Anything deep fried – including fries, fish fingers, chicken fingers, fish and chips
3. Starchy carbs – potatoes, rice, bread and pasta
4. Baked goods – specifically cookies, cake, muffins, doughnuts
5. Soda, juice, and most drinks other than water (coffee is fine, let's not go crazy here)

Breakfast, lunch and dinner dishes are your key to cutting weight. One easy-to-maintain life hack for making this simple system work for me is that I typically don't cook a lot every night.

Rather, on Sundays with my fish dinner, I cook 3 chicken lunches. I put these 3 lunches into separate containers and store them in the fridge to be used throughout the week. Then I only have to cook egg breakfasts and steak/fish dinners on Monday, Tuesday, and Wednesday. While cooking my dinner Wednesday night, I also cook 3 more chicken lunches for the remainder of the week (1 for the weekend). By having all your meals prepared in advance, it will keep you from being tempted with poor choices. In addition, you'll only need to go to the supermarket twice a week. Bonus, right!

I'll just type out a typical week of eating to see if you can handle it

Monday - Egg breakfast, chicken lunch, protein shake (next chapter), steak/fish dinner

Tuesday - Egg breakfast, chicken lunch, protein shake, steak/fish dinner

Wednesday - Egg breakfast, chicken lunch, protein shake, steak/fish dinner

Thursday - Egg breakfast, chicken lunch, protein shake, steak/fish dinner

Friday - Egg breakfast, chicken lunch, protein shake, steak/fish dinner

Saturday - Egg breakfast, chicken lunch, protein shake, steak/fish dinner

Sunday - Egg breakfast, chicken lunch or cheat meal, protein shake, steak/fish dinner or cheat meal. Try to have one cheat meal this day and then back on to the routine.

Once you knock out the 270 meals and you're regularly working out, you'll move to **Advanced Eating**, which will pretty much *allow you to eat anything you want*, as long as it's basically healthy according to our standards. This also includes the odd cheat meal to keep you focused on what you're doing. Cheat meals also keep eating enjoyable and help you not to feel so constricted.

Although we're close, we're not quite there yet, and temptation may come back into play between meals, so let's talk about something really important as we move forward...

Snacking.

14

Snacking – Our Yellow Brick Road

One thing you can be sure of from this plan is that your body will want to snack...and *frequently*. There is a direct relationship between your size and your hunger between meals. The formula goes like this:

If you're bigger→ you'll have a bigger stomach→ which will secrete more grehlin→ which will make you hungrier!

What you need to be able to do is successfully *manage* your expectations with prudent, timely snacking. As per the vitamin section, if you're eating a multi, you won't get cravings for specific nutrients as you'll already have plenty in the tank.

So this positions your snacking habits in one of two negative categories:

Psychological trigger (as in, *"I always munch on something between lunch and dinner..."*)

Or

Caloric deficit

Because we enjoy big, healthy-sized meals, we shouldn't have to worry about the second category so let's tackle the first.

Of course I can't make you read anything that's going to make you stop thinking about snacking, so let's just discuss the types of snacks that **won't hurt your weight loss.**

If you enjoy cooking, and you want to build muscle, one great snack is **cooked chicken strips.** They're the same sized chicken pieces from our lunches and if you make another container's worth just for snacking, you'll be surprised how full just a few high-protein strips can make you feel. Give it a try if you've never done it.

Here's a recipe for a healthy snack that's not just for parties anymore.

Guacamole

4-5 Avocadoes (not too ripe, not too fresh)

1 onion

2-3 tomatoes

1 lemon

1 clove garlic

Halve your avocados, remove the seeds and slice chunks into mixing bowl.

Dice up your onion finely and add it to the avocado meat. Give it a stir to mix them together.

Roughly dice your tomatoes and add to mix.

Clean garlic and slice finely into the mix.

Halve lemon and squeeze juice into mix being careful to remove all seeds.

Add peppers (Jalapeno/Poblano/Habanero if you can handle it) or your hot sauce preference to taste.

Stir it all together and you have some delish guacamole to really give your chicken a kick!

Another snack I enjoy when I'm in a weight cutting period is **almonds.**

I wouldn't get too caught up in which ones to eat (*i.e. roasted vs. raw*) because if you're willing to munch these tasty, guilt-free, healthy treats then you're fine. I sometimes eat almonds at my desk like they're potato chips. This is going to be one of the few times I drop a study on you, but this shows scientifically that almonds are a great snack food in comparison to complex carbs.

http://tinyurl.com/oz28q47

But if I could only have one snack food for the rest of my life, what would it be? *Pez...cherry Pez...*

Actually, it would be **protein shakes.**

Protein shakes are low in carbs and fat while being high in protein. If you've never tried them or haven't had one in years, allow me to assure you that they've made leaps and bounds recently in terms of flavour. Most taste like your favourite milkshake now, even when you only add water. My personal favourite is *Optimum Nutrition 100% Whey Gold Standard – Strawberry Banana.*

http://tinyurl.com/q4okpu7

I strongly recommend getting a 5 lb. container of your fave delivered directly to your home, office, or both! If you had a protein shake every time you got a sugar craving, you would easily and completely satisfy that craving without ingesting the bad stuff.

Now, it must be noted that protein shakes *will* spike your insulin and may inhibit fat burning but, in this case, I'm recommending an exception to the frenemy. Protein shakes provide the perfect link between your main meals without getting you in trouble with refined carbs or candy bars. If you make protein shakes your *go-to snack*, you'll be shedding loads of weight overnight as you'll always feel full.

That's it! That's healthy eating in an almond nutshell. "What?!" you say. "There's got to be more than that!" Remember, I'm trying not to inundate you with an overwhelming list of healthy foods to eat or a ball & chain list to slow you down. It's really very simple: Eat basic foods and *love eating them*.

And please don't think that I'm asking you to eat the same two meals every day *indefinitely*. When you're eating healthy and working out regularly, your eating options will become wide open as long as you maintain common sense. Once you've dropped the weight, feel free to substitute a healthy sandwich for the chicken and veggies at lunch, or a healthy burrito for dinner. Remember, it's not how you get the macros, only that you get the macros. You can even have cheat meals once in a while or sample No-No's like ice cream and pizza (see Advanced *Eating*). For now though, keep your eating clean and your weight loss will progress much faster.

Now, if you're overweight bordering on obese and feel like 1 breakfast, lunch, and dinner won't cut it for now, then just prepare 1 additional lunch and dinner and consume them as snacks between regular meals. Just like with water, you can have as much of this food as you want, and your body will still look to use your stored fat for energy. If you eat like this, the weight will fly off faster than you can buy the new pants which you will need.

If you're in a situation where you feel you might be tempted, make sure you stay one step ahead and stick to your backup snack plan. Personally, I wouldn't even go in a greasy franchise place where they serve something like blooming onions (*the antithesis of eating healthy*) so I wouldn't lose any momentum I've gained keeping the weight off. Your body is a beautiful fat burning machine and you have to give it time to do so. Temptations are everywhere out there of course and you'll need to stick to your guns *and your healthy food* if you want this to work. Remember, you don't always have to say yes to meal invites to disgusting restaurants. There is a power in saying no or offering a healthier restaurant option. After you've lost the weight, we'll discuss more freedom with your food options.

15

Rudy Doodie

Poo. Ah yes...my 2-year old's favourite word and one of our shortest chapters.

Your body is a protein machine. You give it protein, and it gives you life along with the by-products of urine and poo. I hope I'm not overstating the obvious when I say that proper, regular elimination is crucial to losing weight.

When we get into physiology, and more specifically chronobiology, we begin to understand our circadian rhythms and how our healthy bodies want to develop patterns linked to sleeping, eating, and eliminating and so a healthy elimination to start the day is a goal we can all sit down for. Once you begin to manage this for a few days in a row, your body will expect it and your rhythm will be set. A healthy cleansing in the morning offloads all the overnight waste products your body has stockpiled. It also then allows your healthy egg breakfast to get the protein machine revved up, which further sets you up for your high-protein lunch and dinner.

What I do each night before bed is take a tablespoon of fiber with a glass of water. I wake up, I check what's going on online for a few minutes before WHOOOOSH and the bathroom is calling. I am then good for the rest of the day, and don't have to worry about using the disgusting dunnies at my office (they're not that bad, I just hate pooing next to people a few feet away from me, I'm weird). I highly recommend fiber, even if you're not very old.

Now, let's take this to the next level. Have you ever looked at someone and no matter how hot they are, you think that they have a crap on deck in their body? No? Just me? Oh. OK, anyway, have you ever been lying down, and turn over and some gas shoots right to your sphincter to be released? It's because we have these incredible tubes all through us where food and gas can travel or get trapped. By turning your body, you can let gravity help take the food and gases through further. Now stay with me on this. You've probably never thought about it before, but sitting down to poo is not the way we've been doing it for hundreds of thousands of years. Prior to the seated toilet, we were squatting and this is actually the easiest way to poo for the way our bodies are built. In many countries, there are no seats and people poo into a hole in the ground. These countries are known to have fewer issues with diverticulosis and piles in comparison to the Western world. Your body has a number of processes going on to set up a poo, involving two of your sphincters named the internal anal and external anal sphincters. These are working in conjunction with a relaxed puborectalis to allow for a poo to be ready to go. What we are doing when we sit at a toilet is we get ourselves halfway into our natural squatting position. This requires us to push the poo through what is effectively a kinked hose in our bodies. We are squeezing poo through a smaller canal than what it should go.

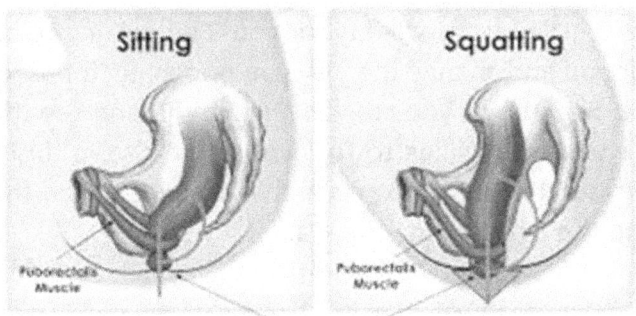

The way to fix this is to raise your legs up when you are on the toilet, kind of like you're doing a cannonball into a pool. You can do this with a little stool for your feet nearby your home toilet, or by simply grabbing your legs when you are ready to poo. This allows for the kinked hose to be straightened and your poo to shoot right out. That might sound bizarre, but once you start doing it this way, it is very tough to going back to that tough old way and giving a mini birth at the toilet each day. Just knowing this trick can change your day, as you know how much a good poo can change your whole mind-set. If you thought that taking one foot out of your underwear was freedom, this will be an out of your body experience (ouch).

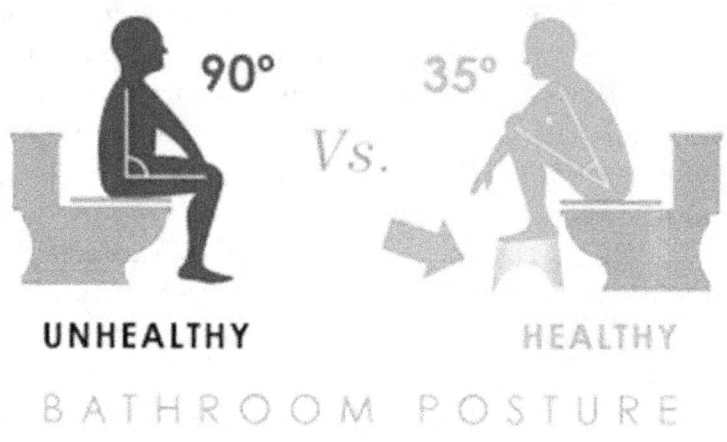

90° **35°**

Vs.

UNHEALTHY HEALTHY

BATHROOM POSTURE

Now, here is a little test of validity for you. I am willing to bet that this will work for you and change the way you poo going forward. Judge my book on this one trick. If you are willing to try it, and see that it works, I think you should be willing to try everything else in this book. But I swear, if this book is only known for teaching the world this poo posture, I will not be a happy chappy. Ha.

16

Accountability Time

Bad news time boys and girls. When you start eating according to the plan, your body will begin to experience profound changes. To put it another way:

You're going to start feeling very weird.

When I started eating this way for the first two weeks I felt like my insides were slowly twisting and turning me into one big knot. This natural phenomenon is your body fully utilizing your stored fat for energy (and in my case for the very first time).

My body was so accustomed to using sugar and refined carbohydrates for energy that of course it was in a state of shock when it had to do otherwise.

This feeling of burning your stored fat instead of your sugar/refined carbs is bizarre and very well may send you straight to the toilet for a bit, but this will be healthy, natural and all good if your overall end goal is cutting weight and feeling better.

The first two weeks are absolutely vital to this eating plan because if you lose faith, break bad and start to cheat/treat, your body won't complete this important flushing process properly.

Be strong in these two weeks, however, and your body will quickly adapt and adjust to deriving its main energy source from healthy foods and you'll be set up for success to come!

Now I have one big favour to ask all of you that are ready to take the plunge and follow my plan:

I want this to be as interactive an experience as possible so I'd like for you to take a photo of yourself in your tightest, clingiest clothing (*less is more*) and e-mail it to my book's site rudysblueprint@gmail.com. Think of everything you've done (or not done) up to now as being your famous "Before" shot.

I'll keep these on file and after your first 90 days, take another one, send it in, and then we can compare the difference.

I've found that sometimes the most effective way of rewarding yourself (and you will deserve a reward) is to look at photos of yourself before you started eating healthy and compare. Then, in the future, whenever you think you've reached a plateau, look at the "old" you.

I know these basic photo memories will help you to push yourself even further.

If you then follow through on your work-outs, we can do an even more encouraging comparison every 90 days. *I'd love nothing more than to be your personal virtual trainer!*

And please *tell everyone* that you're doing this. Not for promotional purposes but because the more people you tell about your new direction, the more accountable you'll feel to yourself to ***make it happen! Gamify the change by posting this meme on your wall. See how many people are with you!***

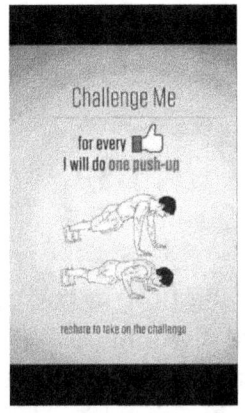

Being a project manager, I'd be remiss if I didn't introduce the latest buzzword into this system. That word is "agile" and I think it can work brilliantly in this context. When you work in an agile manner, you work for 2 weeks and then have a look back at what you've done right and wrong (called a retrospective in IT jargon). For weight loss, you will drive yourself crazy if you look at the scale every day so I suggest you proceed in an agile manner: work for 2 weeks and only check the scale at the end of that time. Then review your progress and analyse where you might have gone wrong and what you can fix. Did you drink sugar water too often? Did you drink too much at your friend's party and wound up out of commission the next day? These things can be pinpointed and not repeated in the next two weeks. This is how you will get better and continuously improve. If you get really good at it, then you should move into software delivery with me.

17

Music

Now instead of my just listing how to cook planned meals and telling you to get it done, I figured it would be a bit more interactive if I listed out 270 songs for you to try whilst making the meals. I feel like a great new song sometimes saves my life when I hear it and add it to my playlist. Personally, I would easily pay the price of this book for a couple of new songs in my life, so think about the value you are getting with 270 to choose from. I'd like to think I'm going to put you on to some obscure bangers but if you know them all, then you know a tiny bit about music like me. Be sure to friend me on social media. I always want to know more like these!

As a disclaimer, I'd like to say that I have not contacted any of the publishers of these songs and I have no connection to any of the groups. I just love their work. If anyone from a group or publisher would like a song removed, I am happy to take it out.

I am not going to write out every link to these songs as they can change over time. I will leave it to you to find how to play them. This is a link to them on my YouTube channel. http://tinyurl.com/q5xzsue

Obviously it helps their cause if you buy the song and play it that way. You can read my first book for my opinion on downloading. Nuff said. If any of these get you going, best to add them to your workout playlist for the next phase of the book. OK, let's get stuck in.

Song	Artist
1. I Can Change	LCD Soundsystem
2. I Love It	Hilltop Hoods (feat. Sia)
3. Spank	The Naked And Famous

4.	Uprising	Muse
5.	Getting Scared	Imogen Heap
6.	New York State of Mind	Nas
7.	Sheila	Jamie T.
8.	Trembling Hands	The Temper Trap
9.	You Know You're Right	Nirvana
10.	Missing Pieces	Jack White
11.	Dreamgirl	Dave Matthews Band
12.	Scream (Funk My Life Up)	Paolo Nutini
13.	Salute	The Diplomats
14.	Machu Piccu	The Strokes
15.	So Appalled	Kanye West (feat. Jay-Z, Pusha T, Cyhi the Prince, Swizz Beatz, RZA)
16.	Breezeblocks	alt-J
17.	To The World	Kanye West (feat. R. Kelly)
18.	I'm Going Down	Bruce Springsteen
19.	In Tha Park	Ghostface Killah (feat. Black Thought)
20.	Zero	Yeah Yeah Yeahs
21.	The Downeaster "Alexa"	Billy Joel
22.	Coochie	Blakroc (feat. Ludacris & Ol' Dirty Bastard)
23.	Hands Of Time	Groove Armada (feat. Richie Havens)
24.	1 Train	A$AP Rocky (feat. Kendrick Lamar, Joey Badass, Yelawolf, Danny Brown, Action Bronson and Big K.R.I.T)
25.	Judith	A Perfect Circle
26.	Girls Like You	The Naked And Famous
27.	Rich Kid Blues	The Raconteurs
28.	Chase That Feeling	Hilltop Hoods
29.	Home	Edward Sharpe & The Magnetic Zeros
30.	Hunting For Witches	Bloc Party

31.	Glad Tidings	Van Morrison
32.	My Doorbell	White Stripes
33.	Thin Line	Macklemore & Ryan Lewis (feat. Buffalo Madonna)
34.	GO!	Santigold
35.	L.A. Song	Deconstruction
36.	Acapella	Kelis
37.	Sail	AWOLNATION
38.	Troublemakers	Ghostface Killah (feat. Raekwon Method Man and Redman)
39.	Lean On	Major Lazer & DJ Snake (feat. Mo)
40.	Footsteps	Pearl Jam
41.	6th Avenue Heartache	The Wallflowers
42.	From Eden	Hozier
43.	Beautiful People	Chris Brown (feat. Benny Benassi)
44.	If You Steal My Sunshine	Len
45.	Something About You	Level 42
46.	Hurricane	MS MR
47.	Song 4 Mutya	Groove Armada
48.	Then She Did	Jane's Addiction
49.	Made in America	Jay-Z and Kanye West (feat. Frank Ocean)
50.	Bam Bam	Sister Nancy
51.	Pressure Drop	The Specials
52.	Tupelo Honey	Van Morrison
53.	Rudie Can't Fail	The Clash
54.	Scarlet Begonias	Sublime (cover of Grateful Dead)
55.	Mercy	2 Chainz (feat. Big Sean, Kanye West and Pusha T)
56.	Runnin'	David Dallas
57.	Beautiful War	Kings of Leon
58.	We Found Love	Rihanna (feat. Calvin Harris)
59.	This Time	John Legend

60.	Excursions	A Tribe Called Quest
61.	Little Black Submarines	The Black Keys
62.	Flagpole Sitta	Harvey Danger
63.	Artificial Life	Operation Ivy
64.	Under Cover Of Darkness	The Strokes
65.	Posse In Effect	Beastie Boys
66.	Oh No	Noreaga
67.	Love Lost	The Temper Trap
68.	Where Are You Going?	Dave Matthews Band
69.	Over And Over	Hot Chip
70.	Fast Lane	Eminem (feat. Royce Da 5'9)
71.	Waiting For Your Time To Come	The Datsuns
72.	I Don't Like	Big Sean (feat. Chief Keef, Jadakiss, Kanye West and Pusha T)
73.	Feel the Love	Rudimental
74.	In A Week	Hozier (feat. Karen Cowley)
75.	Love Interruption	Jack White
76.	North American Scum	LCD Soundsystem
77.	Team	Lorde
78.	Sitting Inside My Head	Supergroove
79.	Madness	Muse
80.	Gold On the Ceiling	The Black Keys
81.	Get Lucky	Daft Punk (feat. Pharrell Williams)
82.	1%	Jane's Addiction
83.	Way Too Cold	Kanye West
84.	Strong	London Grammar
85.	Sister Christian	Night Ranger
86.	Old Enough	The Raconteurs
87.	Africa	Toto
88.	Precious Illusions	Alanis Morissette
89.	Dead Man Walkin'	Bruce Springsteen
90.	Barton Hollow	The Civil Wars
91.	Fascinated	Company B

92.	Clique	Kanye West (feat. Jay-Z And Big Sean)
93.	Self Control	Laura Branigan
94.	Kids	MGMT
95.	Elderly Woman Behind a Counter	Pearl Jam
96.	Jigsaw Falling Into Place	Radiohead
97.	Dancing On My Own	Robyn
98.	Buggin' Out	A Tribe Called Quest
99.	Uninvited	Alanis Morissette
100.	Looking Down the Barrel of a Gun	Beastie Boys
101.	Latch	The Kin (cover of Sam Smith)
102.	Us	Regina Spektor
103.	Hey Mister	Custom
104.	Rap God	Eminem
105.	Skyride	Dead Air
106.	My Friend	Groove Armada
107.	What A Great Night	Hilltop Hoods
108.	Banned From TV	Noreaga
109.	Settle Down	Breaks Co-Op
110.	What's My Name?	Rihanna (feat. Drake)
111.	I Will Possess Your Heart	Death Cab for Cutie
112.	Hey Hey What Can I Do?	Led Zeppelin
113.	Candy	Iggy Pop
114.	Someone Great	LCD Soundsystem
115.	Bones	Giacomo Picasso & Jackson Allen
116.	Things Done Changed	The Notorious B.I.G.
117.	Bad Town	Operation Ivy
118.	Victory	Puff Daddy (feat. The Notorious B.I.G.)
119.	Memories	David Guetta (feat. Kid Cudi)
120.	The Chain	Fleetwood Mac
121.	Pumped Up Kicks	Foster The People
122.	Three Days	Jane's Addiction

123.	All My Friends	LCD Soundsystem
124.	Stimulation	Method Man
125.	White Dude	Lil Dicky
126.	Little Talks	Of Monsters and Men
127.	Knowledge	Operation Ivy
128.	Packin'	Porno for Pyros
129.	Wolf Like Me	TV On the Radio
130.	Finger Lickin' Good	Beastie Boys
131.	Girl from the North Country	Bob Dylan (feat. Johnny Cash)
132.	God Said No	Dan Bern
133.	Bartender	Dave Matthews Band
134.	The Man's Machine	Jamie T
135.	Julie & the Mothman	Kasabian
136.	Give It To Me	Timbaland (feat. Nelly Furtado & Justin Timberlake)
137.	Millionaires	The Script
138.	Stupid Marriage	The Specials
139.	Birthday Song	2 Chainz (feat. Kanye West)
140.	Lateralus	Tool
141.	Gallows Pole	Led Zeppelin
142.	All I Need	Method Man
143.	All Apologies	Nirvana
144.	You're Nobody (Til Somebody Kills You)	The Notorious B.I.G. (feat. Faith Evans & Diddy)
145.	Wagon Wheel	Old Crow Medicine Show
146.	Candy	Robbie Williams
147.	Get It Together	Beastie Boys
148.	Jack-Ass	Beck
149.	Lonely Boy	The Black Keys
150.	You Make Loving Fun	Fleetwood Mac
151.	The What	The Notorious B.I.G. (feat. Method Man)
152.	No One	Alicia Keys
153.	Cannibal	Children Collide
154.	Forever Now	Cold Chisel

155.	Castles Made Of Sand	The Jimi Hendrix Experience
156.	Matchbox	The Kooks
157.	Streets Of New York	Kool G Rap & DJ Polo
158.	Up The Bracket	The Libertines
159.	Nothing Compares 2 U	Chris Cornell (cover of Prince)
160.	Gigantic	Pixies
161.	So What'cha Want	Beastie Boys
162.	Synchronicity II	The Police
163.	Order Of Protection	50 Cent (feat. Lloyd Banks and Tony Yayo)
164.	All I Really Want	Alanis Morissette
165.	Do I Wanna Know	Arctic Monkeys
166.	Looking For Trouble	Kanye West (feat. Pusha T, CyHi Da Prince, Big Sean & J. Cole)
167.	Hurt Feelings	Flight Of The Conchords
168.	Middle of Nowhere	Hot Hot Heat
169.	Sticks 'N' Stones	Jamie T
170.	Runaway	Kanye West (feat. Pusha T)
171.	Bloodbuzz Ohio	The National
172.	Pass The Mic	Beastie Boys
173.	Cold Water	Damien Rice
174.	Tiger Woods	Dan Bern
175.	Gangsta Sh*t	Snoop Dogg (feat. Loon)
176.	Smiles Don't Lie	Thundamentals
177.	Downtown Train	Tom Waits
178.	Dance Hall Days	Wang Chung
179.	Ready 2 Go	Martin Solveig (feat. Kele)
180.	Rattlesnakes	Lloyd Cole & The Commotions
181.	Blue Jean	David Bowie
182.	Like a Version	Illy (covers Silverchair, Hilltop Hoods, Paul Kelly and Flume)
183.	Romeo and Juliet	Indigo Girls (cover of Dire Straits)
184.	Area	The Futureheads
185.	The Hard Road	Hilltop Hoods

186.	Beamer, Benz, Or Bentley	Lloyd Banks (feat. Juelz Santana)
187.	400 Lux	Lorde
188.	The Becoming	Nine Inch Nails
189.	Respect	The Notorious B.I.G.
190.	Aenima	Tool
191.	Mad Izm	Channel Live (feat. KRS-One)
192.	Ashes To Ashes	Faith No More
193.	Root Down (Free Zone Mix)	Beastie Boys
194.	Us Against the World	Coldplay
195.	Eskimo	Damien Rice
196.	Let Me Go	HAIM
197.	Operation	Jamie T.
198.	Substitute for Love	Madonna
199.	Halftime	Nas
200.	Addicted	Bliss N Eso
201.	The Girl You Lost to Cocaine	Sia
202.	Muhammad My Friend	Tori Amos
203.	Until The End Of Time	Tupac Shakur
204.	The Bridge	MC Shan
205.	You Are the Sunshine of My Life	Stevie Wonder
206.	Please Me Like You Want To	Ben Harper
207.	Freestyler	Bomfunk MC's
208.	Let Forever Be	The Chemical Brothers
209.	Paper Romance	Groove Armada
210.	Midlife Crisis	Faith No More
211.	Fuckin Problems	A$AP Rocky (feat. Drake, 2 Chainz and Kendrick Lamar)
212.	A Small Victory	Faith No More
213.	Shadowboxin'	GZA & Method Man
214.	The Nosebleed Section	Hilltop Hoods
215.	Me Plus One	Kasabian

216.	Fairytale of New York	Pogues (feat. Kirsty MacColl)
217.	Wait For You	Tammany Hall
218.	A Sorta Fairytale	Tori Amos
219.	Off The Books	The Beatnuts (feat. Big Pun)
220.	Siva	The Smashing Pumpkins
221.	Caledonia	Paolo Nutini (cover of Dougie MacLean)
222.	Hey Soul Sister	Train
223.	Outer Space	John Grant
224.	Cosby Sweater	Hilltop Hoods
225.	Zombie	Jamie T.
226.	Close Your Eyes	Run The Jewels (feat. Zack De La Rocha)
227.	Happy Idiot	TV On The Radio
228.	Lazaretto	Jack White
229.	This Modern Love	Bloc Party
230.	High	Peking Duk (feat. Nicole Millar)
231.	It Will Come Back	Hozier
232.	El Scorcho	Weezer
233.	Werewolves of London	Warren Zevon
234.	Salt Peanuts	Dizzy Gillespie and His All Star Quintet
235.	Gold	Chet Faker
236.	Forty Six and Two	Tool
237.	Pale Green Ghosts	John Grant
238.	4th Chamber	GZA (feat. Ghostface Killa, Killah Priest, RZA)
239.	Bubble Toes	Jack Johnson
240.	Back To Earth	Rusted Root
241.	All Gold Everything Remix	Trinidad James (feat. TI, Young Jeezy and 2 Chainz)
242.	The Golden Path	The Chemical Brothers
243.	Lover Man	Charlie Parker
244.	Radio	Santigold
245.	Alloway Grove	Paolo Nutini
246.	Days of Fire	Nitin Sawhney

247.	Candy's Room	Bruce Springsteen
248.	BROOKLYN	Young M.A. (feat. Rell Markz and LA Danger)
249.	Definition	Blackstar
250.	Molly's Chamber	Kings of Leon
251.	No Diggity	Chet Faker (cover of Blackstreet)
252.	Street Riders	The Game (feat. Nas and Akon)
253.	Geronimo	Sheppard
254.	Common People	Pulp
255.	Best Friend	Yelawolf (feat. Eminem)
256.	Murder She Wrote	Chaka Demus & Pliers
257.	Empire	Bomb The Bass (feat. Sinead O'Connor and Benjamin Zephaniah)
258.	New God Flow Remix	Kanye West (feat. Pusha T and Ghostface Killah)
259.	Take Ecstasy With Me	Chk Chk Chk (cover of Magnetic Fields)
260.	Silvergun Superman	Stone Temple Pilots
261.	Little Black Box	Stan Walker
262.	Are You Old Enough?	Dragon
263.	Ride A White Horse	Goldfrapp
264.	Teardrop	Massive Attack
265.	Maynard's Dick	Tool
266.	Banquet	Bloc Party
267.	Lucky Man	The Verve
268.	Koko	Charlie Parker
269.	Whiteman in Hammersmith Palais	The Clash
270.	Every Other Freckle	alt-J

"The downtown trains are full with all those Brooklyn girls,

they try so hard to break out of their little worlds.

You wave your hand and they scatter like crows,

they have nothing that will ever capture your heart.

They're just thorns without the rose,

be careful of them in the dark."

-Tom Waits "Downtown Train"

18

The Ween

Reading wise, you are now at the official halfway point of the plan. If you've spent the 90 days on the quality food, you should be seeing dramatic results.

You may think this is only halfway along the path or that maybe you're only halfway there or only won half the battle. But let me tell you something important right here and now:

If you're now eating healthy, you've already won. You don't even need to do the rest because the Ween is for those who want to see how far they can push themselves.

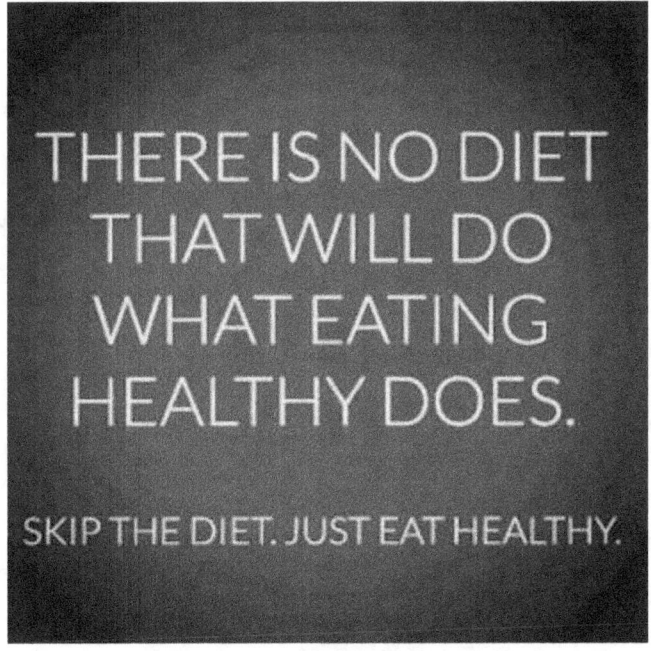

THERE IS NO DIET
THAT WILL DO
WHAT EATING
HEALTHY DOES.

SKIP THE DIET. JUST EAT HEALTHY.

If you've been eating properly, you should be well on your way to feeling great and looking even better so, at this point, I'd like to take a moment to explain to you the other big secret that fit people aren't always anxious to share.

It's called **portion control.**

Portion control is a huge factor for your sustained health and once you successfully practice its simple secrets, you'll not only shatter that psychological dependence on giant-sized meals but you'll also feel fitter, faster and be amazed at how well your body works with the proper amount of fuel. Yes, less will be more once again!

So, *starting right now*, begin to limit your meals to smaller amounts. You'll discover that your body can handle these portions much more efficiently than the larger meals (with all the trimmings).

Starting from **your very next meal**, your steak should be *no more than 130 grams (5 ounces)*, your chicken should be *no more than 250 grams (9 ounces which basically equals 1 breast)*, and let's cut back to *3 whole eggs in the morning (but still as many egg whites as you like)*. If measuring food isn't up your alley, just think about your meat portion not being much bigger than a pack of playing cards.

In addition, use the size of your fist as a guide to dole out your vegetables.

The Ween is another key to your sustained health. It's a way for you to discover that your body is indeed an awesome high-performance engine and you're its best mechanic.

If you don't feel like working out, just try the Ween for 90 days. When you've finished, let's get a photo of you in front of that mirror you'll never need to avoid again. Send it to rudysblueprint@gmail.com and we'll compare the results.

If you now want more results, then here we go...

19

We're Gonna Work Out

An Introduction

This is the first chapter of many on working out (or "training" for my non-US readers).

Again, this book is meant to be read sequentially so you should be reading this chapter *only* if:

You're eating clean and healthy (as per previous instruction).

You've dropped the excess weight (as per previous instruction).

To reinforce those previous instructions – *and to ensure that all you line-jumpers out there get it right this time* – let's be clear on one thing: If you radically change your eating habits *and* try to start any type of serious work-out program *at the same time*, the enormity of the task will cause you to

Give up working out, give up eating right, or both.

You need to make eating healthy your numero uno priority before you can even think about working out. Here are some reasons why.

Your eating habits will give you 70% of the results you want and need. Working out will cover the other 30%.

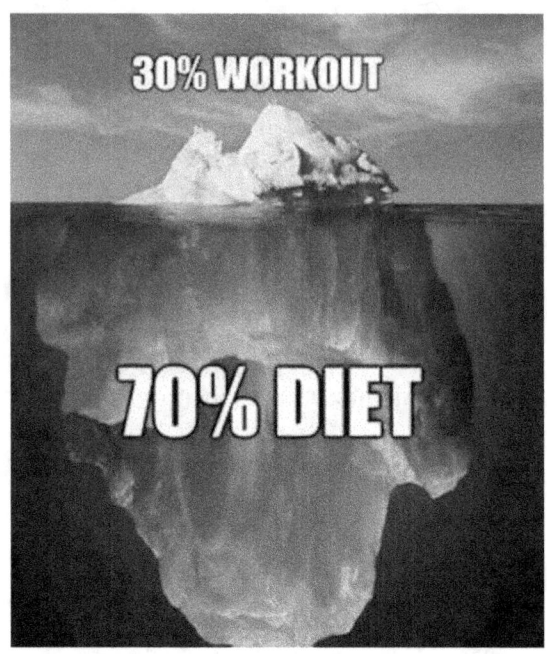

When you attempt to work-out while overweight, the fat you haven't lost yet will mask any muscle gains. As a result, you will not see results in the 3 months needed for this section.

Working out with weights creates microscopic tears in your muscles that heal and, over time, increase the size of those muscles. Your body weight, however, should not, and must not, tear your muscles.

This is why you need to *eat right first to lose the weight.*

I believe in the idea of baby steps for this big change so let's ease you into working out and start off with *bodyweight exercises* first. After you've mastered these, you can get into a gym to do some *free weight work.*

But remember, you do you.

If you're content with just the bodyweight exercises, then just stay in that zone until you can safely progress. The last thing anyone wants is to get injured. Always move forward at your own pace.

For these next chapters, you'll see a number of website links. I can assure you that these are all thoroughly researched and worthwhile. I've researched hundreds, if not thousands, and these are the cream of the crop (feel free to message me on FB or Twitter if any links are down).

If anything, I'd like you to understand that this "working out stuff" is a *science*. So please read even more than what I suggest if you feel it helps.

So...are you eating healthy?

Grrrrrrrrreat! Now let's move on.

20

Common Workout Misconceptions

Before we dig in let's first cut the bullshit and dispense with some of the most common workout misconceptions out there that may have held you back in the past.

I can do enough just walking or running – Negative. Walking doesn't do much besides slightly increasing your heart rate. The muscles involved in walking alone *do not* become sufficiently stimulated to burn enough calories to cut weight. In addition, 1 cup of coffee will negate a brisk 30-minute walk.

Running is slightly different as it *does* burn more calories, but still not enough. A 5K run burns about 400 calories which is the equivalent of half of 1 muffin. Suffice it to say, dancing around to music will give you no results, although it might be a good laugh. Pushing weight with proper form is what will get you there. With weight training, your body burns calories even at rest, and for days, as it's rebuilding your muscles. Think of weight training as a great *compound interest plan* for your body as it works even while you sleep.

I need to join a gym to work-out – Ridiculous. You can get a full body workout at home or in a park without a single piece of equipment. There are countless creative ways to stimulate every muscle in your body without joining a gym.

I need to spend hours in the gym every time I go – Nope. Work-outs should be limited to *45 minutes at most*. Anything more than that and your results are in decline. The aim is to tear the muscle and replenish your body with the food needed to repair it.

No Pain, No Gain – Please. You don't have to torture yourself to get a great body and your workouts don't need to be masochistic. Training your muscles effectively can easily be accomplished without insane pain.

I need to sweat a lot to get a full workout – Wrong. You don't need to sweat one drop in your quest for a great body. When you work with weights and concentrate on simply training muscle groups gradually – and finishing properly – you should not need to break a sweat. I will explain this further later.

As a woman, if I work-out with weights, I'll get bulky – Nonsense. I've heard this one from women afraid of getting big: *"I have a big ass, so I don't want to make it bigger."* This is, in fact, totally the opposite of what would happen. If, for example, you did happen to pack some extra gear in the rear and you then did squats/ lunges/leg uplifts, you'd only make it *smaller and tighter.* The muscles involved would feed off the fat to sustain itself. And fortunately for women, you *do not and cannot* create enough testosterone to get bulky, period.

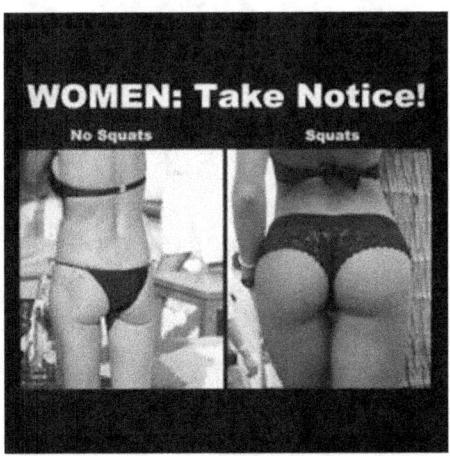

I'll Need To Eat 6 Meals A Day – Another myth. *Total caloric* count is what matters most in a day, so whether or not you get it from 6 meals, or 3, it will affect you the same.

21

The Buy-In

Managing Your Expectations

I'll personally never look like a fitness model and I'm fine with that. What you may think these models are isn't really all that close to reality when you consider how much they fast before photo shoots. They'll even cut out sodium and water to get "the shot." In the long run, this type of deprivation isn't sustainable.

I don't believe every man aspires to look like a fake-tanned, muscle-bound freak in a budgie smuggler. I've never wanted to look like a barrel-shaped power lifter who looks like he can bench press a cow but might have big problems scratching his back.

Let's be realistic with what you want to do with your body. So which morph are you?

http://tinyurl.com/5u94we

If you're a tall and naturally thin person, an *ectomorph*, you'll find it harder to stack on serious muscle. That being said, tall and thin is a great look with defined muscles. Any of the morphs are a good look with defined muscles. None of us are going to be – *and most of us don't want to be* – body builders, so why judge yourself by other people's standards. Just be the best *you!*

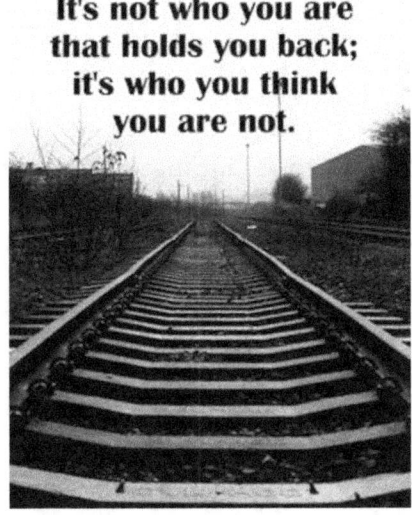

**It's not who you are
that holds you back;
it's who you think
you are not.**

Another thing that people don't fully understand about the body is the limits to what you can do without steroids. I've heard about football players in the offseason packing on 20 pounds of muscle and it always makes me go "hmmmmm?" That is not physically possible without cheating. No matter how good your training and legal supplementation is, your average gains can only really get to about half a pound of muscle a week. So keep in mind that muscle gains are a slow process, but well worth it.

I do not work-out for a living but I can help you get to where you want to be. What I would really like though is for you to develop a genuine passion for working out and eating right. If you can catch *that passion*, you can easily surpass any goals you may have thought were out of your reach. If you want to really get into it, you should "like" fitness pages on Facebook and Instagram, get e-mail updates about nutrition and weight loss, and continually seek out the things that motivate you. As for me, I have no problem viewing ripped models on fitness sites because it makes me get off my ass that day and *do something*.

You only have 365 days until this time next year. What are you doing NOW towards being a better you?

Let's begin.

Body Weight

For the beginner, you need to get intimately acquainted with your body weight. Because you've been eating healthy and shedding the weight, you can get a terrific workout with just the weight you're carrying right now.

One thing I want to stress in this chapter is that you will never look better than when you can repeatedly lift your own body weight. I know a lot of girls who think their arms will get freakishly big if they do triceps workouts, dips, or push-ups. This is pure nonsense. If getting big were that easy, all guys would be freaking huge. If you can pull your body weight up, or push it off the floor continuously, you *will* get *very lean* very quickly but not big. You only get big by lifting weights heavier than what your muscles normally handle. A woman doing multiple push-ups, pull-ups, or dips, would develop a physique like *Linda Hamilton* in *T2*. Developing a physique like her male co-star would require lifting lots and lots of heavy weights (not to mention drugs).

I find it easier to work-out at a gym because just getting there focuses my effort. I think it is akin to studying in the library as opposed to your dorm room (when you're in college, of course). Consequently, these chapters will prepare you for the gym. Having said that, one thing you can do easily at home is *circuit training.* This is when you do one set of an exercise, then a different set followed by another. You can get a whole circuit of different sets in and then rest. At the gym, circuit training can become problematic but I'll get to this later.

There are viable ways to work-out without going to the gym. Herschel Walker made his transformation from fat kid into superhuman by doing 5,000 push-ups and 5,000 sit-ups every day. I'm not asking you to do anything close to this but it is a good example that you don't need any weights or machines to get work in.

Here is a breakdown of what to do for each main body part:

Push-ups

Chest and Triceps – Begin with 20- 30 reps

Push-ups are the best exercise you can do for your chest. I'll repeat that again.

Push-ups are the best things you can do for your chest. *And you can do them anywhere you go!*

Simply place your hands in front of you and then on the floor.

Straighten your body from your shoulders to your legs while staying on your toes (you should look like a perfect plank).

Keep your body locked and let your arms depress you to the ground.

Touch your chest to the ground.

Push back up to the starting position.

That is 1 push-up.

If you put your arms farther out, you work more of your chest. The closer you place your hands together, the more you work your triceps. I do 50 push-ups before my shower each morning. It's the best way to wake up your body after a night's sleep and it really gets the blood going.

Air Squats

Hamstrings, Quads, and Glutes – *Begin with 20-30*

Squats are the best things you can do for your legs. Shall I repeat that? Yeah why not. **Squats are the best things you can do for your legs.**

Begin with your legs shoulder-width apart

Slowly drop your bottom to your ankles

Push back up.

I usually extend my arms in front of me for balance. If you can do this easily, do 20 of them. Then do more than 30. If you can get up to over 50 of these in a row and do 4 sets of them, you may want to look into a gym membership because your legs are in fantastic shape already. Women tend to store fat around their hips and thighs. This is natural. In order to trigger further fat burn of these areas, more blood needs to be going through them to turn fat into energy. Air squats are a great movement for that. Another great one for your bottom is donkey kicks. Look them up.

Pull-ups

Latissimus dorsi, Biceps – *Do as many as you can.*

Pull-ups are the best things you can do for your back muscles. And just for my OCD side of things, I'll repeat it. **Pull-ups are the best things you can do for your back muscles.**

You can usually find a bar to hang from in any park near your place. If you want to do them at home, you'll need a pull-up bar for your door-frame (sold at any gym store). This movement is pretty basic but it's one of the hardest to do.

Grip the bar firmly with your hands shoulder-length apart

Pull your body up until your chest almost touches the bar. Hold this position for a second.

Lower yourself down.

Please note how I ask you to hold yourself when you get to the top of the movement. This 1 second hold on each rep will have an exponential effect on your results.

If you can do one of these, that's awesome.

If you can do 10 of them, move onto 15 and then 20. If you can do 20, start looking at gyms. If, however, you're struggling with the first one, simply move a chair underneath you, grip the bar, and use the tips of your toes to push off of the chair. I know how hard the first one is but once you get past it, you'll be addicted.

After you can do 2 or more, feel your lats after a week or so and see how defined they start to get.

Bicycle Crunches

Abdominals and obliques (also known as your core) – *Do 4 sets of 20*

Working on your abs only makes sense if you're eating right. If you have a big belly going on, you're pissing in the wind when you do ab work. But let's assume that you've been eating right. **Bicycle crunches are all you need for ab work.** It is the most effective movement you can do for your core. Your core is a set of muscles that can recover very quickly so they can be worked on every day and between sets of other exercises. The brilliance of the movement is that you get the *north/south* action that you'd get from a standard crunch, as well as the *east/west* action that you'd get from a *Russian twist*. This is how you do it.

Starting Position:

Lie on a mat, with your lower back pushing against the floor (this helps with your TVA).

Put your hands on either side of your head by your ears.

Bring your knees up to about a 45 degree angle.

Movement:

Slowly go through a bicycle pedalling motion alternating your left elbow to your right knee then your right elbow to your left knee.

Fully extend the leg not being brought to your elbow and keep it low to the ground.

Key Points:

Do not perform this activity if it puts any strain on your lower back.

Do not pull on your head and neck during this exercise.

The lower to the ground your legs bicycle, the harder your abs have to work.

The key is to breathe out every time you contract your ab muscles. That is how the muscles get tension.

Perform this exercise in a slow, controlled fashion for sets of 20.

Men tend to store fat in their bellies and love handles. To lose the love handles, you need to get blood going past them to turn the fat into energy.

Resistance Bands

I picked up resistance bands for my home gym. While I thought they would just help out on a couple of muscle groups, I've come to find that, when used properly, they can be used for *all muscle groups*. Try these if you plan to work-out primarily at home. The logic behind them is pretty basic: *You're doing muscle movements with tension on them.*

Links:

7 minute bodyweight workout:

http://tinyurl.com/q6oswzj

44 body weight exercises video:

http://tinyurl.com/b59p82f

I particularly enjoyed these articles:
http://tinyurl.com/o694dxu

http://tinyurl.com/po65few

http://tinyurl.com/pw23s2t

http://tinyurl.com/pgasvwb

http://tinyurl.com/p7sflwp

Here's one of my favourite, simple, everyday routines:

Begin by doing push-ups and air squats in the morning before your shower. Do 20 air squats and as many push-ups as you can (up to 50).

Find a pull-up bar and do as many as you can (up to 10).

If you do these every morning, weekends included, you'll see results within 2 weeks. You will also have the blood flowing and will be so much more awake and invigorated.

Do more of these sets at night and throw in bicycle crunches (up to 20).

This is a good routine for those of you who go on business trips and stay at hotels with subpar gyms. You don't need the gym, you can work-out in your room.

When you're comfortable doing all of these exercises, as in:

50 push-ups in one go

20 air squats in one go

10 pull-ups in one go

20 reps on each side of slow bicycle crunches

Congrats! Now it's time to move to the next stage and join a gym.

22

Uncommon Common Sense

Look...If you like running, then *run*. I don't want to be lumped in with the naysayers so if you decide to start running instead of sitting on the couch, as we say down here:

"Fill yer boots!"

It's not that I consider running as necessarily a bad thing, it's just that I know squats can give you a better result in a fraction of the time. If you can do *HIIT* (High-Intensity Interval Training) go right ahead. If we even briefly compare the bodies of sprinters to long distance runners...well, HIIT works! And If I'm near a set of monkey bars when I take my daughters to the park, I do 10 pull-ups because every single pull up begets another one. This is how **muscle begets muscle**. In short, any activity that moves you towards working out will lead to *more working out* and gets a big YES from me. When it comes to getting fit, something is always better than nothing!

Love Working Out

Another confession that I'm happy to make:

I love working out.

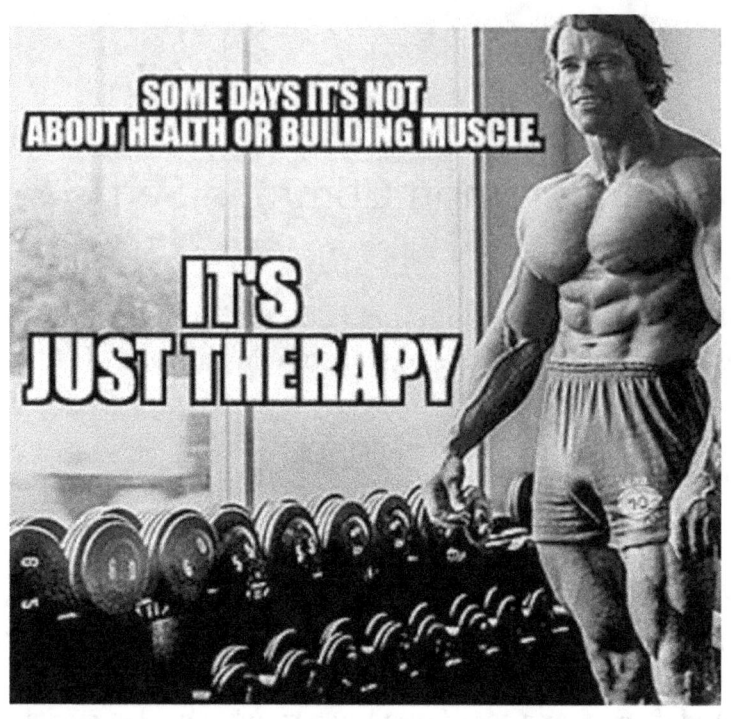

I love the results and I love seeing myself get stronger, adding reps, and seeing – and feeling – myself get tighter in the mirror. I love feeling the groove in my sternum from tightening my core and I love the way my days and weeks feel complete when I get all of that excess energy out of my system.

Another big reason why I love working out, is that *I love eating...a lot!*

Muscle begets fat burning because it always takes more calories to sustain muscle than to sustain fat. So when you get muscular, you're setting yourself up for weight loss because your body will be working hard even when you aren't thinking about it.

The gym is my temple away from work. When I'm working out, I forget about all my problems, worries, and stressful thoughts. My workout time is my "Me" time. I meditate, zone out to music, and forget about the day and all the random craziness in my life.

And of course, it's pretty easy to see that creating a toned body will make you more physically attractive to a prospective partner. Let's face it...a girl with defined shoulders, legs and a sweet ass is so much hotter than a girl with flabby arms and a saggy bottom. We all know it's the same for guys. Females are genetically, evolutionarily designed to be more attracted to a fit man rather than to a fat one. But while it's nice to work-out to impress others, in time, you won't be working out for anyone other than yourself.

When you choose to get into working out, you'll quickly arrive at a point where you'll feel that if you don't do something athletic each and every day then you're doing your body a grave disservice. Getting to this point is very, *very good!*

To this end, I believe you should start working out 3 days a week with a target goal of moving to 4-5 workouts a week. Muscles are usually fully healed in just 72 hours so after 3 days, don't be afraid to put them through the wringer again. Believe me, when you feel one of your biceps and it feels like a ball peen hammerhead, you won't want to stop.

I believe a person's body can be a great reflection on their life. People that have their bodies in order usually move on to keeping *everything else* in order. One simple but profound change can start a stampede of changes for the better. And I know that all it takes is *your lunch hour.*

Your Lunch Hour and its Treasure of Time

I've been "lucky" enough to be able to work-out on my lunch hours for the last few years of my career. The reason I write "lucky" is because I work damn hard, and I know my work's management is willing to let me go every day, as long as I keep it up. I know this because I am part of management as well, and I give my high performers a long leash. Your lunch hour is the secret treasure of time that can give you all the rewards you're seeking and much more.

Of course most people use their lunch hours to have a breather, play games on their phone, smoke a cancer stick or sometimes even go for a walk. Coming from someone who used to use the last option I can state that, after a while, your neighbourhood will become stale, you'll end up bored, or worse (for your wallet at least) you'll go shopping. I know some people who don't bother going out at all and just eat at their desks. This is the worst choice. Don't chain yourself to your desk and don't allow anyone else to either. If your job requires this, you may want to look for other work.

Staying at your desk allows you no respite from your job, gives you no perspective, keeps you stressed and is ultimately counter-productive.

I tend to see people at lunch walking around, contemplating the banality of living this ridiculous circus ride of circling the sun 75 times and flying towards a black hole in the Milky Way. OK, maybe they just look like they're thinking this but they do look like they're walking around aimlessly and wastefully. Instead, we should be, *and could easily be,* making the hour work for us!

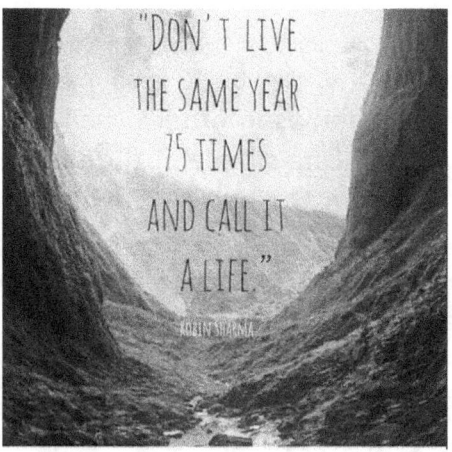

Instead, I ***strongly suggest*** going to the gym at lunch. Break up your day and help yourself out!

I only work-out for 30-40 minutes at lunchtime, and then I eat my lunch at my desk afterward. If you can find a gym near work, I suggest you make it happen!

As an example, here's my typical lunch schedule:

12:00 – Leave the desk, go into the changing room.

12:05 – Changed and walking to gym.

12:10 – In the gym, and onto my first set (mapped out ahead of time).

12:40-12:45 – Finished and leaving the gym.

12:50 – Back in work dressing room suiting up.

12:55 – At my desk enjoying a post workout protein shake.

Later, around 2-3PM, I put my high-protein lunch into the microwave and fuel up.

Boys and girls, it can be done. Be clever.

Let me explain something about the lunch hour workouts: **You just gotta go.** Maybe make a sign saying this, and don't even think about not obeying. Just get there, get through it, and move on. Sometimes just getting there is the hard part but even a half-ass workout is better than no work-out. Sitting in the gym is better than sitting at your desk. Once you can rationalize not going, or only going 3 times a week, it's a slippery slope.

I'm always one step ahead. After breakfast, I know I have a workout coming up in about 5 hours. I run the kids to school and day-care, give my job its requisite attention, and then, at 11:45, start preparing for my workout with a bit of pre-workout nutrition in the form of PRE and a protein shake.

During my workout, I consume a BCAA drink. And then after my workout I have another protein shake. I work a bit and then have lunch at 2:30 or 3PM. I do my afternoon work, and then have dinner at 6:30. Basically, my daily activities – including my job – revolve around my workout.

As for people who feel they don't have time to exercise, I get it. But I also know this:

At my various work places, I've had colleagues who never miss a daily workout, and I've had colleagues who never bother to work-out at all. I can't say that the ones who exercise are better at their jobs than those who don't, but I *do know* that the gym rats have just as much going on in their lives. We're talking about busy people with similar jobs and similar family situations.

Your body is more important than your job. Notice I didn't say that your workout is more important than your job. Obviously some work things can't be missed, but you should not prioritise your job before your body every work day. You need to hit that gym. **You need to get it in.**

So it's not about the time, it's about what you want to do with your time.

Personally, when I'm tempted to skip a workout, I remind myself that I've never regretted exercising but I always regret *not exercising*.

No Stretching and No Sweating

As you've probably noticed, my lunch schedule allows around 35 minutes for a full workout. Needless to say, I do not waste time stretching... and I do not sweat at all.

I know that sounds a bit strange but I changed my body within 6 months to building the type of muscle I want, to benching 400 lbs(up from 300 lbs), and getting a 6-pack without wasting time stretching and **without EVER breaking a sweat.**

Here is a pic of my wife and me in Hawaii, after 6 months of working out 4-5 times a week, without sweating, still drinking alcohol and doing only bicycle crunches for core.

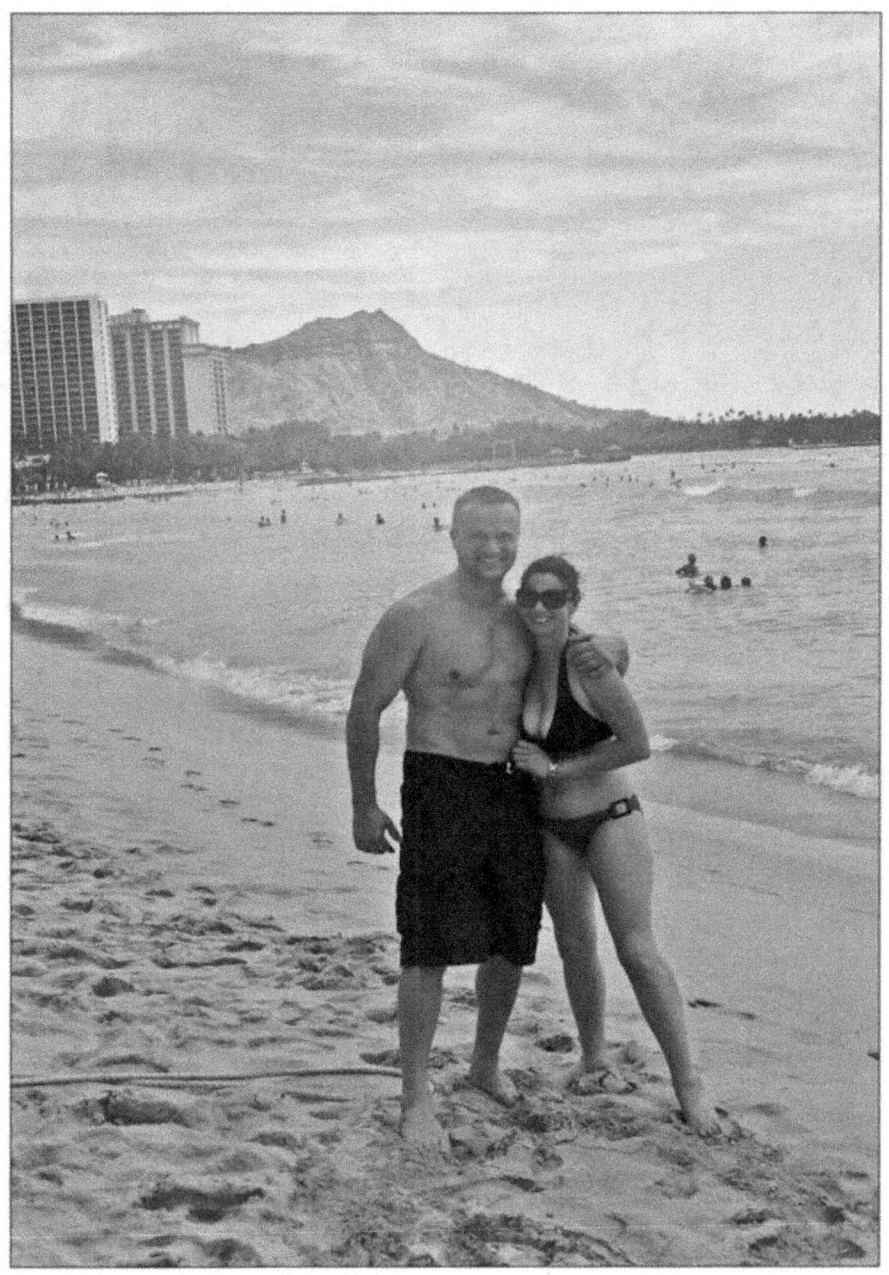

And this is 12 months later, in Fiji, without drinking alcohol (huge difference in core) for that same period but with more intense ab exercises, still no sweating.

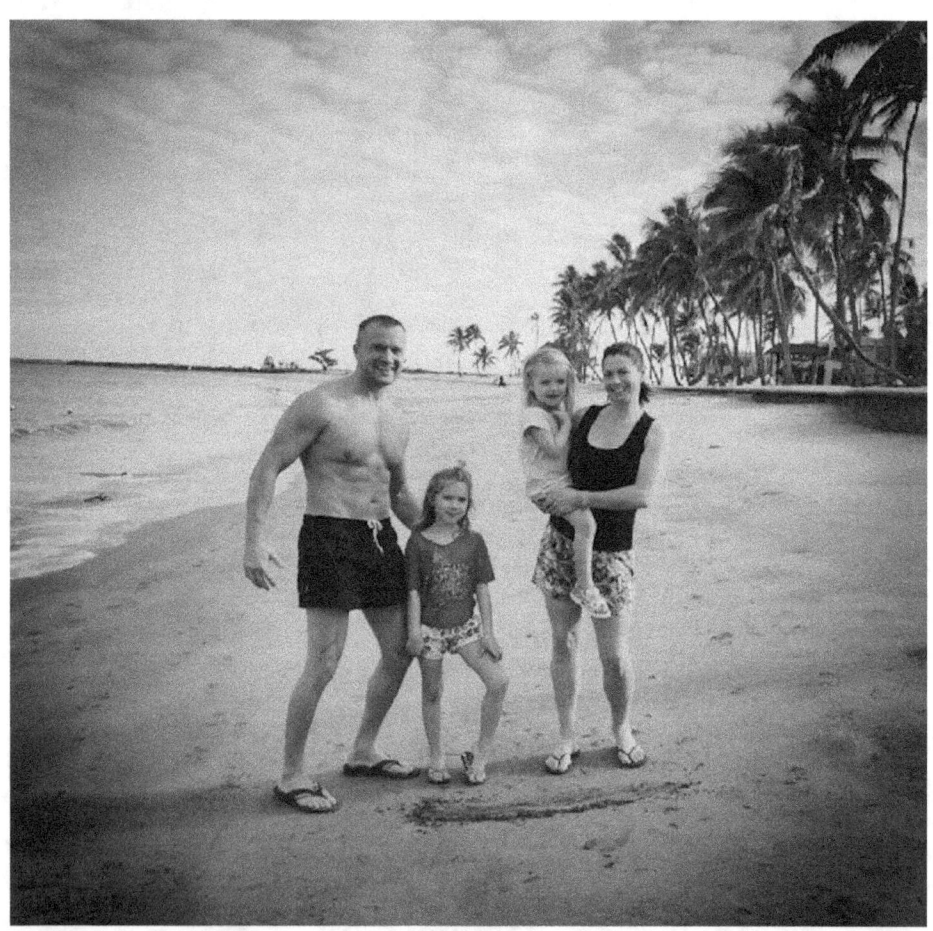

12 months later with supplements, no alcohol, eating more for mass and no sweating.

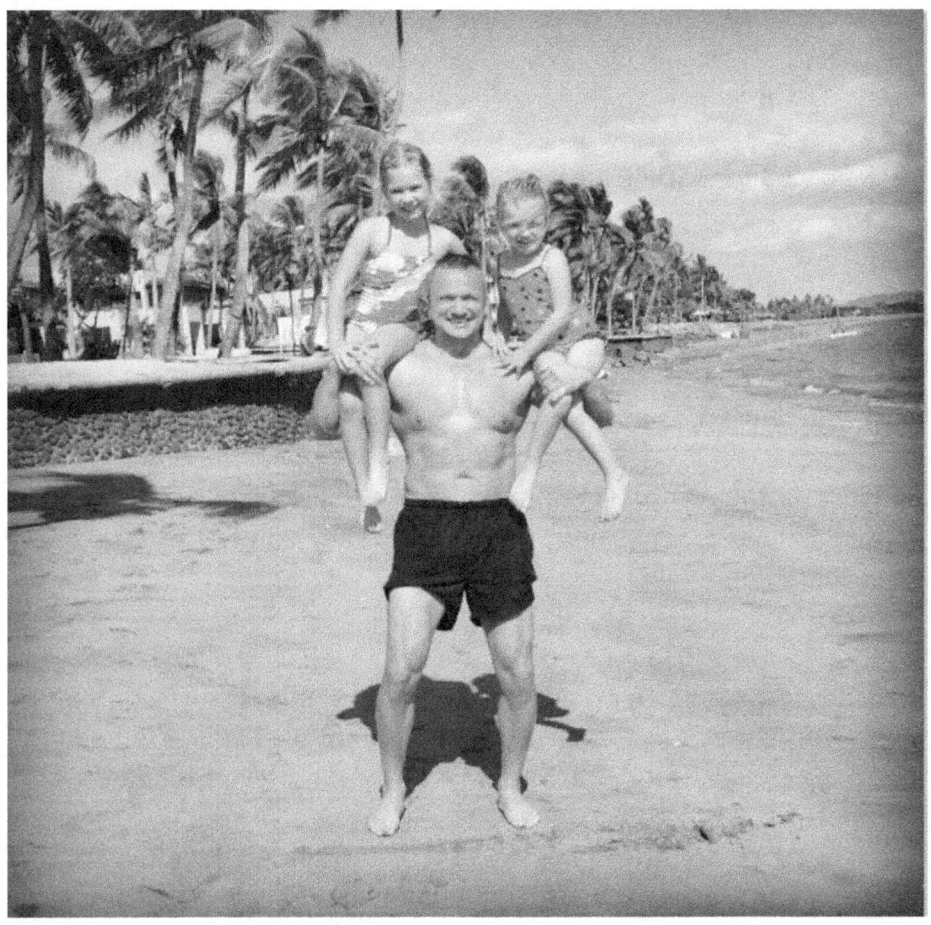

Supplements: with consistent weekday work-outs, and this eating plan, they work. And Dadbod? Whatever. Don't be like the sheep.

Please believe me when I say – *ANYONE can do this! Now it's your turn.*

Now if I spent any time stretching, it would eat into the precious 35 minutes so I make my first set of the day the time for a gradual *stretch* to loosen up.

For example:

For back and biceps, I'll do a set of pull-ups without any weight.

For chest and triceps, I'll do a set of bench presses at 50-60% of the weight I'm aiming for in the next sets.

For legs, I'll squat 50-60% as well.

If you take your time and move with purpose, you'll be stretching sufficiently while you're working out. Of course stretching out on a mat feels good, but it's never been conclusively proven to enhance your workout. For this plan, time is of the essence. Get your stretching done *while you're working out!*

And just for the record, I maintain good flexibility (I can easily place my palm on the ground without bending my knees and I can scratch my upper back if needed).

Now, if I had to shower a second time after each workout due to sweat, it would slow me down by about 5-7 minutes. Time is crucial during the lunch workout so I like to save that 5-7 minutes. I also don't like the idea of carrying a wet towel back to work and home each day.

I work-out each day strictly with weights, no cardio. I'm not totally against cardio, but the amount you need to do (45 minutes for 300 calories) is wasteful. It also eats away at your muscle mass. There is, of course, a time and place for cardio, and that is *the weekend* and done via *HIIT:*

http://tinyurl.com/7nrgvo6

The microscopic tears are how your muscle builds and the simple fact is that you don't need to sweat to tear muscle. So even if you aren't limited in time, you simply don't need to be drenched in sweat after a workout to get muscle definition.

Am I telling you to do weight training alone?

No, but if you only have 5 minutes to change into workout clothes, 30-40 minutes to work-out, and 5 minutes to change again, it's still not only possible but very manageable to do weight training alone and still get and keep a body that is, *"Toit as a toiger."*

Even if you do go to the gym before or after work, you should limit your workouts to 30-40 minutes there. Once you start spending an hour or more working with weights, you're in "overkill" territory. Overkill territory can actually work against you because you need to start healing your broken muscle fibers rather than putting more wear and tear on them.

Don't get me wrong, I still do a Latvian shower — *deodorant spray* — when I change back into my work clothes. No doubt, my co-workers are pleased that I do.

Having a limited amount of time to work-out makes you push harder to fit it all in. If there's no time limit, beginners tend to get lazy and end up giving up. Stay busy and active. Keep your mornings and nights free to live your life, not work-out.

23

Uncommon Common Sense – The Gym

Joining a Gym

When I started searching for my current gym, I wanted one that was very close to work and had dumbbells that weighed more than 88 lbs (40 kilos). That might not be a deal breaker for you, but I needed more weight than this for my chest and back work. I saw two gyms before I found one with dumbbells that go up to 130 lbs (60 kilos). Awesome.

You may have other criteria when looking for a gym. Things like friendly staff, opening hours, clean facilities, classes, or even good-looking people can make or break a gym for some people. I'm not too social at the gym and actually prefer to just zone out with my iPod and work-out like no one is there. I've made the odd acquaintance here and there, but I never spend more than 40 seconds talking to others between my sets. My strict words of advice at the beginning stages: *Don't let anyone slow you down.*

I lucked out with my latest gym as it's fairly new. It has new equipment and a good, cheap monthly rate to attract customers. If you can get new equipment with a decent rate, go for it.

12-month contracts are usually standard but I wouldn't do 24 months as you don't know where you'll be 2 years from now for work. I usually do a 12-month plan and pay monthly after that period if I'm still there.

The link below is a fascinating article about joining a gym and actually making use of your membership. The business model for most gyms is that they want to make money on the basis of members that pay, who *actually fail to go*. By going each lunch hour, you would be way ahead of the curve of the unmotivated.

http://tinyurl.com/n354u3z

Another thing to look for in a gym is the amount of equipment. I say this because nothing sucks more than a gym with only 1 bench or 1 squat rack that people are lining up to use.

You might want to ask them what their peak times are and try to avoid them. For example, if they peak at noon each day, you might want to take your lunch at 11:00AM or 1:00PM. Peak times mean fewer choices for you and more people in your way. Monday night is usually the busiest night for gyms around the world because people are trying to start the week off right. You might want to avoid this time if at all possible.

Trainers

Another thing to avoid is the "free" personal training session. This is often just an easy way for their house personal trainers to create a bond with you and then give you the hard sell for 12 or more sessions at a crazy rate.

Here's a good article about bad trainers:

http://tinyurl.com/qdrrbhx

If you need a class or a trainer to make you do something at a specific time, maybe self-motivation is something you need to look into. The fact is that most members hire trainers for socialization and motivation but *you don't need a trainer.* **You can be your own trainer!** Just do it!

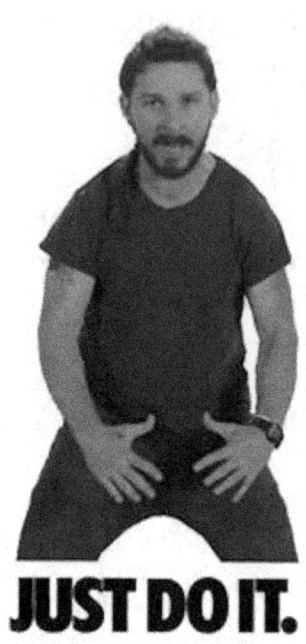

JUST DO IT.

Once you get a routine going to the gym, it will be much harder to not go. Ultimately, it's your call, but I never use them.

That being said, always try to be friendly to the staff — *you may need them to spot you* — and be generous with the nods and smiles to other members. Everyone's going for the same reason so you don't have to feel any different from them, no matter how you or they look. Do you know what I mean? Anybody at the gym has at least made the decision to go there, so why look down your nose at anyone, even if they are large?

So you've joined the gym. Now what should you bring when you show up?

What to Pack

You'll need to wear loose, comfortable, breathable clothing when you're doing the zero-sweat workout. I wear a basketball jersey (no sleeves) because if I do start schvitzing (sweating), the sweat evaporates quickly.

I also wear board shorts with a cargo pocket, to hold my key card for work. You need to wear socks and sneakers, too. Gyms are pretty anal nowadays about wearing sneakers, as they give some protection to your toes if weights fall on them. So don't wear flip-flops, and for God's sake, don't wear Birkenstocks. You're not a Brooklyn hipster and this isn't a hemp picnic. Rest assured that if you waltz in with beat hippie feet, you will be hated like one.

You do *need* to bring a towel. You should be putting the towel on the part of the exercise machine that your head/body rests on. If you forget your towel and you leave head spots behind on machines, you need **to clean up after yourself** with spray (if they have it), or use your shirt or shorts to wipe off.

As far as other workout attire, forget it.

If you're new to the gym, or even if you've been going for a while, you don't need weight gloves or a weight belt. These are both just gimmicks and they make newbies look like fools. And if you think a weight belt is somehow going to miraculously hold your spine together if you try to squat too much—wrong, think again.

As I said above, I bring an iPod to the gym. I'm a music freak and I prefer my playlists over gym music. I'm not there to make friends (even though you end up making acquaintances there if you go at the same time every day), and I don't particularly care if it looks antisocial. Talking to others for too long slows you down, eats into your precious time and is ultimately counter-productive (this is true at work, too). I need music to pump me up sometimes for sets and I like to be able to choose what I want. An iPod isn't critical but if you have to listen to the same crap music being played over the gym speakers at each workout, you will slowly go mad.

Now that you know what to pack, we come to an important question:

How should you act at your gym?

How to Act (and How Not to Act)

Working out is a bit of a tribe-like ritual where it is absolutely essential that you *give a little and you take a little.*

For example, when you get into a machine or bench, just bang out your 3-4 sets in a few minutes...then *move on!*

Don't ask to "work in" with someone. No one likes that, wants that, or wants to hear that. If someone just happens to get a machine or bench before you, just do something else until it's free.

And try not to do two separate exercises across the room from each other. Nothing is more annoying than waiting for someone to come back to a machine because they are trying to superset with a piece of equipment half a room away. Just do your business in one place...then *move on!*

Also try not to bogart multiple pairs of dumbbells. Keep to 1 pair and, again, do your sets...then *move on!* Leave the supersetting for when the gym is empty (my favourite time).

Always take weights off of bars after you use them. It's not proper etiquette to leave the leg-press machine loaded up with 8 plates on each side. Oh, and it does not make you look tough. *Always put dumbbells back after you take them off the rack.* Some people think they can just leave a wake of used weights behind them for the attendees to clean up. That is the equivalent of walking around your office throwing files onto the floor for someone else to pick up. **Don't be that guy!**

The other people in the gym notice this crap quickly and will learn and remember to despise you. *You don't want that!*

Think of it this way: When you take the weights off of bars or walk dumbbells back to the rack, you're putting tension on your shoulders, arms, core, and legs. You're working out while you're cleaning up. This is a *bonus workout* and will actually enhance your results. Every extra rep or weight movement you do is getting you closer to where you want to be.

The same goes for dropping the weights onto the floor. ***Such a newb move!***

Over time it can damage the weights. Also, anyone who feels the need to announce that they did a set by dropping weights is, as my boy Kenny says, a *total wanker*. You'd never see a seasoned gym vet do this. Get the extra work-out by easing the weights down to your lap or the floor. Always try to keep the weights under control. It will help over time.

So now you know how to respect the gym and the others there. Let's get to the meaningful part: The Work!

24

The Work – Part 1

How to Get a Great Work-Out

Let's discuss precisely what you're doing when you train with weights.

By putting your muscles under the stress of weights, you're creating microscopic tears in your muscle. This tearing is an important step in the muscles getting bigger and stronger. Your body works to heal these tears (with that flood of aminos!), and what is created over a long time is a larger muscle group. It can take months to increase muscle size and definition via hypertrophy so if you're not looking to get big muscles, do not fear. *Your body will only get as big as you let it with the amount of weight you use and the protein you put in throughout the day and night.*

If you regulate both to your needs, you'll still create and maintain an amazing body with toned muscles. Once you feel the tears in your muscle, *do not work through it.* Work on another muscle group. Often, for example, when you do squats, your hamstrings can feel like a guitar that just broke a string. That's a good time to put the weight back and let the muscle group heal for a few days. Some bodybuilders on websites talk about doing 30 sets (a set= a *group of reps*) for legs or other parts. Well...*Ermm*...no.

Think logically. You're trying to get the tear and then heal up. Once you feel the tear, you're done with the reps so don't keep pushing it.

When I write about doing 6-8 repetitions (reps), this means you lift and lower, or move the weight 6-8 times. **This is a key concept in working out with weights.**

Here's a good article about reps:

http://tinyurl.com/qduvkg2

As you'll read in the article, you want to be maxed out by the last rep.

How do you find your weight range?

Simply choose a lighter weight, and if you get to the 8th repetition and it feels like you could easily do 3 more than *increase the weight for the next set*. When you find the right weights, you should be able to do at least 6 reps during a set but struggle to finish the 7th or 8th rep. As you get stronger, you should increase the weight as it starts becoming easier.

If you can get your head around increasing weight as you get stronger over the coming weeks, you will easily master working out.

Any gym instructor can tell you that certain muscle groups work together on movements. There is a concept of *push and pull workouts* that I find instructive. The muscles involved in **pushing** something would be: *chest, triceps, quads, lateral and medial delts.*

The muscles involved in **pulling** something would be: back, biceps, rear delts, traps, hamstrings and forearms.

If you do the upper body on the same day, you can gain efficiency as they can all rest for a few days without being reactivated with other exercises. We want to be efficient in the gym and get out quickly, so let's start off with the basic pairings.

Back and Biceps

*Lattisimus dorsi, trapezius (*lats and traps) and *biceps* (bi's) – This started off as my favourite workout pairing growing up because I could gain the attention of the ladies by subtly putting on a gun show (flexing my biceps).

What I didn't know then was that the biceps are a very small muscle group considering the other muscle they're actually partnered with: *the back*. Focusing more on your back is an efficient way to kill two birds with one stone: Your back can always benefit from a bit more attention (because it's a bigger muscle group) and your biceps will be worked in the process.

Chest and Triceps

As my body filled out a bit more after college, these 2 muscle groups became my favourite because a barrel chest was always a hit with the ladies. I was a bit naïve then, but damn it looks good in the mirror and while flexing your chest (by yourself of course). Also, if you know your Latin, *bi* means 2 and *tri* means 3. So if you want bigger arms, you can get them faster by working your triceps because there are more muscles to build. As per the above grouping, if you focus on your chest workout your tri's will be activated and worked in the process. Efficiency!

Legs and Shoulders

Hamstrings, quadriceps, gluteus maximus, and gastrocnemius (hammies, quads, glutes, and calves) and *trapezius and deltoids* (shoulders). Now that I'm middle-aged, I've come to love my leg workouts most. Your legs are probably the most fascinating body parts because there are so many huge muscle groups that are significantly stronger than any others. When you start working out for yourself and not for others, you'll begin to enjoy the burn from leg workouts. They're your own little secret and make your body a lot more symmetrical in the mirror. So learn to love your leg workouts.

Guys like asses and girls like asses so we should all be doing squats and lunges.

With all the focus on legs, it's easy to neglect the other muscle group in this pairing. If you're a guy, strong shoulders will announce your physical presence, which will cause women to feel safe/protected/attracted around you. It's nature at its finest. If you're a woman, well-defined shoulders look ridiculously hot to guys. So don't forget your shoulder workouts! (Legs and shoulders are 2 muscle groups that do not really help each other out when lifting, but they need to be done, so they're usually done together.)

Ways to tell everything you need to know about a guy:
1. How he treats his mother
2. How serious he takes leg day

Core

Abdominals and obliques, rectus and transverse abdominus, and *internal and external obliques.* An easy way to attack your abs is to fire off a set between each set of the other exercises you're doing that day. Keep in mind that, abs can be worked every day because they're a small muscle group that heals rapidly. If you're not using weights, you're not making the microscopic tears, so look to add weight if you can. Again, use common sense. If they're in pain one day, give them a day off.

25

The Work – Part 2

The Routines

You may wonder about other muscle groups such as your *lower back, rear delts, forearms*, and others. These get worked out while you're doing the other groups. When we move on to "Advanced Exercises" we'll devote more attention to them but for now, let's keep it simple and get into a routine.

Another thing you'll notice is that I'm only putting in basic and safe movements in this routine. You may be thinking, "Where are the deadlifts or squats?"

Deadlifts and squats require a strong core and a higher level *gym IQ*. Let's try them and the others a little later on.

For this routine, start off with the trifecta of **3 workouts per week**.

These are the days and groups:

Monday: *Back and Bi's*

Wednesday: *Chest and Tri's*

Friday: *Legs and Shoulders*

If you can't do these days, then pick days that work for you. Try to leave a day of rest in between them in the beginning because you may be sore the day after a workout (your microscopic tears healing themselves) and we want to keep you focused and coming back to the gym. Too many workouts in the beginning will definitely turn you off.

You may wonder why I split the workouts as I did. Most newbie weight lifters work the chest on Mondays so I always make sure to work another muscle group at that time. I don't like waiting for benches.

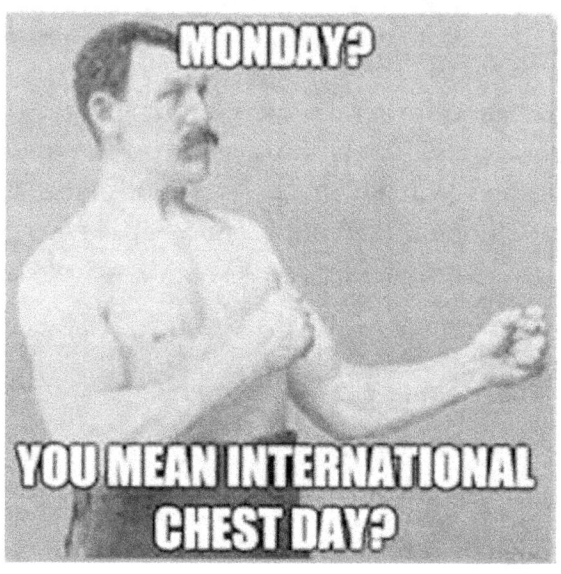

Back & Biceps

I've outlined two routines below. These are to be done *once a week* at first and then *twice a week* as you progress with your number of workouts. You should do *number One the first week* and *number Two the second week* so that your body doesn't get used to the same movements. If you're doing 2 of these workouts a week, do number One on day 1 and number Two 3 days later.

If you work-out 4-5 times a week, you don't necessarily have to start with these over the other groups. You can choose to do legs first which will give you 2 leg workouts a week. This is up to your discretion.

Back & Biceps Routine 1

Pull-ups (as many as you can, for 4 sets)

Standing dumbbell bicep curls (3 sets of 8 reps)

Dumbbell bent over single arm rows (3 sets of 8 reps)

Hammer curls (3 sets of 8 reps) ** *Hammer curls create great forearms as the brachialis and brachioradialis extends around the elbow.*

And then if you have 10 minutes left over:

Chin-ups (3 sets of 8 reps)

Great link for chin-ups. Charles Poliquin is the man

http://tinyurl.com/oebea2e

And don't forget to do your *ab work between sets* (see the Abs section of this chapter for sets and reps).

Back & Biceps Routine 2

Seated Rows (3 sets of 8 reps)

Standing close-grip curling bar curls (3 sets of 8 reps)

Pull-ups (as many as you can for 4 sets) ** *This stays the same; they're the equivalent of squats for your back.*

Standing curling bar curls with overhand grip (3 sets of 8 reps)

And then if you have 10 minutes left over:

One-arm concentration curls or "Arnolds" (3 sets of as many as you can)

Lat Pull Downs (3 sets of 8 reps) ** *Pull to mid-chest*

And don't forget to do ab work between sets.

Here's some great basic exercises for your back that you can work in when you want to switch it up:

http://tinyurl.com/pxk5dj7

Here's some basic exercises for your biceps and forearms:

http://tinyurl.com/prxw2w3

Here's a great article about bicep training:

http://tinyurl.com/q7hurex

Chest & Triceps

As with the Back & Biceps routine, these are to be done *once a week* at first and then *twice a week* as you progress with your number of workouts. You should do *number One the first week* and *number Two the second week* so that your body doesn't get used to the same move-ments. If you're doing 2 of these workouts a week, do number One on day 1 and number Two 3 days later.

If you work-out 4-5 times a week, you don't necessarily have to start with these over the other groups. You can choose to do legs first which will give you 2 leg workouts a week. This is up to your discretion.

Chest & Triceps Routine 1

Flat bench dumbbell press (3 sets of 8 reps)

Close-Grip Dumbbell Press (3 sets of 8 reps)

Incline bench press with dumbbells (3 sets of 8 reps) ** *Many regard this as the best overall work for your chest.*

Triceps Pushdowns (3 sets of 8 reps)

And then if you have 10 minutes left over:

Decline bench press with barbell (3 sets of 8 reps)

And don't forget to do ab work between sets.

Chest & Triceps Routine 2

Flat bench dumbbell flys (3 sets of 8 reps)

Dips (as many as you can for 4 sets)

Incline bench flys with dumbbells (3 sets of 8 reps)

Overhead extensions (3 sets of 8 reps) ** These target the bulky long head muscle, which is the most visible part. This is a must have movement for your arsenal.

And then if you have 10 minutes left over:

Decline bench press with dumbbells (3 sets of 8 reps)

Triceps kick-back extensions (3 sets of 8 reps)

And don't forget to do ab work between sets.

Here are some basic exercises for your chest that you can work in:

http://tinyurl.com/lngjcwn

Here are some basic exercises for your triceps that you can work in:

http://tinyurl.com/nay3yns

Legs & Shoulders

As with the previous routines, these are to be done *once a week* at first and then *twice a week* as you progress with your number of workouts. You should do *number One the first week* and *number Two the second week* so that your body doesn't get used to the same movements. If you're doing 2 of these workouts a week, do number One on day 1 and number Two 3 days later.

If you work-out 4-5 times a week, you don't necessarily have to start with these over the other groups. You can choose to do another muscle group first which will give you 2 workouts for that muscle group each week. This is up to your discretion.

For your shoulders, it is important to try to get 4 *different types of movements* going. You want to do an overhead push movement, a side arm-raising movement, a front arm-raising movement, and a bent over reverse fly. These last 3 highlight all sides of the deltoids. You really want to start off light for this muscle group as a lot of weight isn't needed and this area is prone to injury.

Legs & Shoulders Routine 1

Dumbbell squats (3 sets of 8 reps) ** *Hold a heavy dumbbell in front of you by your chest, legs wide and go as low as you can and back up.*

Seated dumbbell military press (3 sets of 8 reps) ** *Again, start light.*

Seated quad leg extensions (3 sets of 8 reps)

Side arm dumbbell raises (3 sets of 8 reps) ** *Lighter weight and get your elbows above the dumbbells when you raise them for the real burn.*

And then if you have 10 minutes left over:

Seated calf extensions (3 sets of 8 reps)

Seated or face down leg curls for hamstrings (3 sets of 8 reps) ** *These are great for your ass.*

And don't forget to do ab work between sets.

Legs & Shoulders Routine 2

Dumbbell lunges (3 sets of 8 reps) ** *I usually do these walking the length of the gym. You can do these with just some space in front of you if you lower and then raise back to your starting spot.*

Front arm dumbbell raises (3 sets of 8 reps)

Hamstring curls (3 sets of 8 reps) ** *Usually, the leg extension machine doubles for this movement, but I prefer the lying down ones on your belly.*

Dumbbell bent-over reverse flys (3 sets of 8 reps)

And then if you have 10 minutes left over:

Standing calf extensions using a machine (*Smith machine, donkey press, et al.*) (3 sets of 8 reps) ** *For a better burn, try one leg at a time with half the weight of your regular calf workout.*

And don't forget to do ab work between sets.

Remember that for all the workouts, *time is of the essence.* You want to do as much as you can as fast as you can *before* you leave the gym. Don't waste too much time recovering or socializing. Every rep is better than not doing a rep.

Here's some basic exercises for legs that you can work in:

http://tinyurl.com/odxzb5z

Here's some basic exercises for shoulders that you can work in:

http://tinyurl.com/oo3k3c3

Here is the routine in a table format:

Monday	Tuesday	Wednesday	Thursday	Friday	Saturday	Sunday
Squats	Bench Press	Pull Ups	Lunges	Flat Bench Dumbbell Flys	Seated Rows	
Military Press	Close-Grip Dumbbell Press	Dumbbell Bicep Curls	Front Dumbbell Raises	Dips	Curling Bar Curls	
Leg Extensions	Incline Bench Press	Bent Over Rows	Leg Curls	Incline Bench Dumbbell Flys	Pull Ups	Take A Break, Recover and Recharge
Side Raises	Tricep Pushdowns	Dumbbell Hammer Curls	Bent Over Flys	Tricep Kickback Extensions	Curling Bar Curls Overhand Grip	
Standing Calf Raises	Decline Bench Press	Chin Ups	Seated Calf Raises	Decline Bench Dumbbell Press	Arnolds	
			Abs Done Every Day			

For anyone who can't remember a plan like this (called a push/pull/legs split) I suggest copying this into Excel and adding in a few columns to tick them off as you go.

Abs

Abs are usually today's primary fitness standard. Great abs are like the guy's version of great tits. If you can see them, it tends to make people think you're lean and also that you work on them and on your other muscle groups equally.

So what makes this particular muscle group so special?

In order to get these muscles to really pop, you need to be quite lean, which means it's imperative that you maintain a *very healthy diet*. With your abs, it's usually the last place the fat drops and, conversely, *the first place that you put it back on*. Maybe that adds to their mystique. There are anomalies of younger people eating crap and still having great abs but over time, when their metabolism decreases, their abs disappear if their diet doesn't improve.

Abs are a relatively small muscle group, and the workouts for them don't necessarily need to involve any more weight than your body weight. In fact you can work them with your body weight *every day* as they recover very quickly in comparison to other muscle groups. If you start adding weight to the workouts (later chapter), then they should get the proper rest period that your other muscles get.

For now, all you need to concentrate on is the Bicycle Crunch. Throw in at least 4 sets of 20 reps (to start) while you're resting between other exercises.

Here's some more helpful information about your abs:

http://www.bodybuilding.com/fun/lisa3.htm

Now Do More!

This may seem quite obvious but if you can get through all of the above and still *do more*, then by all means...***do more!***

Don't leave anything in the tank, get it all out. You should be trying to excite your muscles as much as you can. Only bodybuilders need real rest for body parts. You're not one, and neither am I. Do a set of dips on the way to the locker room, do some pull ups in the playground with your kids. Bonus points for doing some walking lunges on the way back to work or throwing in a final few pull ups. It all counts. Your last rep in every exercise will decide how you want to look.

Are you pushing your limits? *Or are you playing safe?* It's all on you.

NOBODY CARES, WORK HARDER.

Keep pushing yourself. It will continually make you crave more action and get you to your goal quicker.

I also love to have a goal in mind when I'm working out. My wife usually plans trips 4-6 months in advance, and I work-out with these trips in my mind. If my next trip is to Fiji, I keep that in my mind when I'm training or saying no to drinks or to eating shit. A goal with a set date can save your butt. When you reach the goal, and take the photo, you'll be in a great place to set your next goal.

Techniques to Avoid

It's naïve to think that every workout technique you've seen is actually effective. If done improperly, any movement can cause more harm than good. Obviously any movement can be done wrong, but some of these movements are considered good ideas by novices. Let me tell you – *They are not good ideas! Don't do them.* Here are some workout no-no's.

Upright rows – This is a textbook technique that you see in movies or TV shows. Try this movement with a broomstick and you'll immediately notice that it puts your deltoids (tops of your shoulders) in a rather odd position. It's this position that makes the Upright Row a bad choice. The Upright Row causes your shoulder to rotate internally and puts unnecessary stress (impingement) on a tendon that can result in long-term damage. *Stick with the shoulder workout that I provided above and avoid the risk.*

Bench Dips – Traditional bench dips are done by facing away from a flat bench, placing both hands on the edge behind you, and then lowering and raising from there. This movement is similar to the Upright Row in that you're internally rotating your shoulders and opening them up to serious injury. It's much better to *use parallel bars* for this movement. Most gyms offer these for use.

Behind the Neck Shoulder Press – These are bad for the opposite reason: you're *externally* rotating your shoulders. Just like internal rotation, external rotation exposes your shoulders to the possibility of injury. Keep any overhead presses happening from the side, or in front of you, and remember to *stay light* in the beginning. Novices tend to think their shoulders are as strong as their chests. *This is never true!*

Behind the Back Lat Pulldowns – You may be seeing a pattern here. Don't do any motions behind your neck. Only do lat pulldowns *in front of your chest.*

Smith Machine Squats – Squats are only for advanced training but I've seen these done by newbies. The Smith Machine is the piece of equipment where you lift the bar, turn it to unlock it from the rack, then move it in a rigid straight line. It seems like an obvious machine for squats because you don't need a spotter but ***this is not the case.*** The brilliance of a squat is that it forces you to balance up, down, side-to-side and front-to-back. It hits basically every leg muscle by making you maintain your form. The Smith Machine takes the side-to-side and front-to-back balancing out of the equation and only allows for you to concentrate on up-and-down balance. This *creates unnecessary strain on your knees and lower back* which can result in an injury. Just say *no* to the Smith Machine...for everything.

Pre and Post Workout Nutrition

I hate to be the one to break it to you, but if you kill it in the gym and then go out and eat crap, you're doing it wrong.

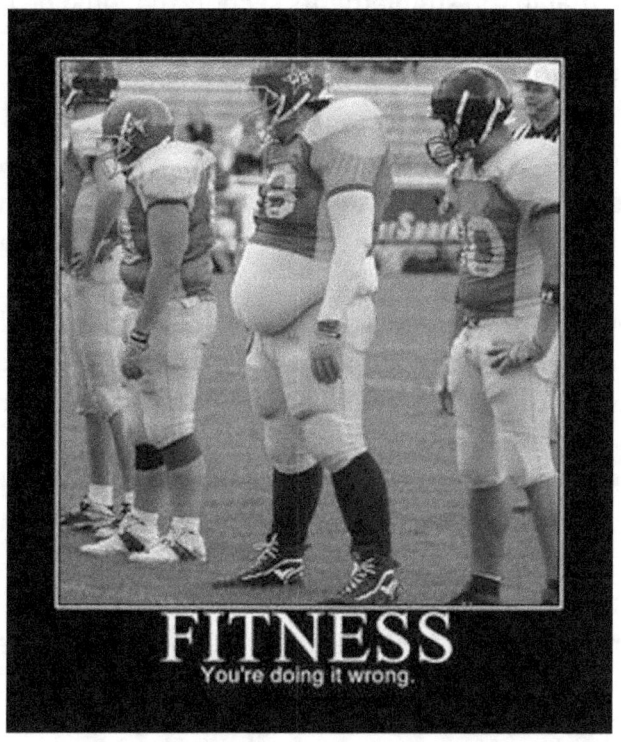

As I mentioned earlier, we're currently living in a brilliant time – The All Access Information Age. We know it's foolish to think that we really know *anything* about the universe, but at least we know more than even 20 years ago. So let's work with that.

What we know *now* is that a workout is *maximized during the peri-workout period*. This is just a fancy term for the time before, during and after a workout.

This is where Insulin is now your *friend*.

Pre-workout: Drink a one scoop whey protein shake around 15 minutes prior to your workout. I put Optimum Nutrition PRE in with this, but I'll get to that in the supplements section. It would be good around this time to eat some carbs from a sweet potato as well. This is a fast acting carb food that can give you energy for your workout

During the workout: Drink a shake of BCAA's, which are just amino acids (discussed further in Supps section), and flood your body with these as they get taken straight to the muscles you're working on.

Post-workout: Drink a whey protein shake with a spoonful of glutamine powder immediately after your workout. I then also eat all my starchy carbs for the day, so sweet potato or potatoes or brown rice all get eaten within 30 mins at my desk. Then 90-120 minutes later (the protein shakes should keep you full until then), consume a high protein (*chicken, lean steak, turkey, fish*) and veggie meal to seal the deal.

I like to think of my pre- and post-exercise protein shakes as "bookends" for my workout. If you're super serious about seeing results, these 3 drinks (before, during, and after) will get you there.

Whey is a quickly-digested protein source that is a by-product of cheese manufacturing. Remember Little Miss Muffet? After your workouts you want to flood your body with amino acids to repair the muscles you just slightly tore. Whey quickly increases muscle synthesis.

The way to look at the carbs is to think about what you need to perform a hard workout (heavy lifting). You are burning carbs, so you need carbs. You need them to start the workout off and give you that energy boost, and then you need them when the workout is over, to replenish your energy stores, and shuttle the aminos to the parts that just got worked. But think of your body as a car. If you drive it slow and easy for only a few miles and then stop to put in the normal amount of fuel, the tank is going to run over because you didn't use very much fuel during your drive. If, on the other hand, you put your car through its paces (i.e. drive it fast and hard for many miles), the car will definitely need fuel or it will stop running. Your body is no different. If you aren't really killing it in the gym and you top up with carbs, your tank will runneth over and lead to sugar in the bloodstream and all the negative effects that involves. If you give it your all, your body will use the carbs to keep you going rather than release them into the bloodstream.

It's absolutely imperative to increase your carb and protein intake around your workouts. You're simply not maximizing your workouts if you're not doing this. This is a secret of those in the know but I want to let you behind the curtain on this one.

For the best results:

Pay as much vigilance to your peri-workout nutrition as to the workout itself.

And if you've never paid peri-workout nutrition too much attention, you're really in for a treat when you start.

26

The Pump

Let me assure you of something: There is nothing cooler than seeing results. If you do nothing but follow my advice thus far, you're sure to see some excellent results. If you've done all that and are hungry for more results, read on.

That being said, this is another check-in moment.

I only want you to look into the following chapters if you're hooked on working out and have been doing so for at least a few months.

Asking an out-of-shape newbie to do a squat is not fun for anyone involved...especially the newbie. So if you still feel a bit unsure about yourself, *reread and redo* the previous chapters until you raise your gym IQ and your body feels good and ready.

Ready for some advanced stuff?

Let me start by giving you some quick insight into my training.

I once spent 12 weeks adding 100 lbs to my bench press to see if I could go from 300 lbs (136 kilograms) to 400 lbs (181.5 kilograms). I got the idea from Tim Ferris's book *The 4-Hour Body,* and I can't believe I'm saying it, but it actually worked! I even had a group of people around me on the final lift in week 12 (I needed 2 guys spotting anyway). The foolish part about it is that each chest workout over the 12 weeks would wipe me out in about 10 minutes. My muscles were being ridiculously torn each week and I felt like puking after finishing each set.

My point is that this is *not sustainable.*

Working out now, for me, is not really about maxing out each time then feeling like crap. It's about setting goals, reaching them, and moving on. I now work-out with "heavyish" weights that will accomplish what I want them to accomplish without leaving me crying next to the bench. I'd rather look good and *feel good* as opposed to benching the most in the gym. There's a school of thought that if you are benching the most at your gym, you're in the wrong gym, because you need people to look up to. But do what works for you because how you view working out is your own individual choice.

Now let's get a little deep and do a comparison in our heads. Think about the strength of two trees, one growing indoors and one outside in the elements. *Which do you think would invariably become strongest?*

The one outside, of course, because it's being put under different strains, stresses and all types of uncontrollable conditions. *And it's the same for your body.*

You *should be* varying your workout routines every day. You don't want to get stuck performing the same routine twice a week, every week because your body will "learn" these limits, adapt and adjust to the minimum requirements for that routine, and then plateau.

A truly fantastic feature of progressing in your training and knowledge of your own body is that when you apply yourself over time, *you'll effectively do much more with much less.*

So I'm going to begin this part of the Plan by introducing you to compound sets that hit a number of muscle groups at the same time. By doing *sets* of these sets, you'll be doing 2-3 groups simultaneously. This will wear you out quicker but also shorten your workouts. Both very good things.

Advanced Exercises

Back & Biceps

Deadlifts – If you look at Hugh Jackman's workouts, he's not polishing off the guns with concentrated sets, he's doing compound movements like deadlifts. Deadlifts are pretty much a full body movement. If you're serious about training, they need to be a staple in your routine just like pull-ups and squats. I've saved them for this section because you should have a strong core before attempting them. I've learned to do them in my socks as the weights get heavier so I have more stability under the bar. You'd be surprised how much your sneakers give you dangerous height for this movement.

Check out these sites for form:

http://tinyurl.com/o6men3t

http://tinyurl.com/q84rb76

http://tinyurl.com/nqha76x

Curls (21's) – 21's are 3 sets of 7 curls for your biceps (hence the name). While standing, do a set of 7 reps from your chest to halfway down. Then immediately (with no rest) do a set of 7 reps from your legs to halfway up. Finally (again with no rest), do a set of 7 reps with full range of motion (from your legs to your chest). Fair warning, these KILL! Obviously, you can't go too heavy as you want to do a high number of reps, so be smart. Always start light if you want to practice. This is a great article on 21's:

http://tinyurl.com/o97ekmp

And this is a further article on biceps training:

http://tinyurl.com/q9tvqze

Pull-ups – I'd also suggest that you buy or use a dipping belt (not to be confused with a weight belt, which is useless) and do weighted pull-ups. These are gold for back training. Also, try doing pull-ups where you go toward one arm instead of straight up. This gives much more of a range of movement for your back as well.

Chest & Triceps

Flat Bench Barbell Press – This is a great compound movement that utilizes your chest, triceps, delts and more. When done properly and in combination with dumbbell presses and flys, it can add great depth to your chest. Keep in mind that these can also be done incorrectly and lead to all sorts of trouble (of the "self-guillotine" type).

This article discusses the history and mechanics of the press:

http://tinyurl.com/q2gukp2

Skull Crushers – I like these for the full feeling of hypertrophy in the triceps. I do about 6-8 with a weight that burns then I do a quick 8 reps of close grip chest presses.

Great video of them here:

http://tinyurl.com/lhxjdca

Legs and Shoulders

Squats – What can I say about squats? When done correctly, they're the best things you can do for your legs. Certain "bro science" trainers will say that they even enhance your production of testosterone but that is a myth. You get a testosterone boost because you are working out large muscles. This is a great article on the squat:

http://tinyurl.com/phzh8bp

And this article explains that the back squat is not for everyone:

http://tinyurl.com/qznsdwd

I personally love front squats and dumbbell squats, but that's just me.

Calves – As previously stated, the most lopsided look is the chicken leg one with a big upper body. You need to get your tree trunks swoll, and the calves are a big part of this look. The key to these guys is repetition, not in the number of reps, but more along the lines of doing them every other day if you can. Use the various ways to push weight off of them taking into account that straight, standing leg calve lifts will affect the gastrocnemius muscle (which is the upside down heart shaped one we normally see) and seated calve raises will hit the soleus (which is the one that runs underneath it, felt if you bend your knee during a calf raise). The gastrocnemius gives you that definition and the soleus gives you the width needed to look in proportion.

This has a great visualization of leg work-outs and each muscles hit on each movement (brilliant!):

http://tinyurl.com/otvj7sf

Shoulders – Defined shoulders on both men and women are a great look. They really make a person look like they know about working out. Anyone can do bicep curls or pushups and be a faker, but shoulders and traps show that you mean business.

Check out this article on the Shoulder Shocker:

http://tinyurl.com/pxe2qpt

Here's a complete guide to shoulder training:

http://tinyurl.com/qftk54j

Supersets And The Next Level

This is another behind the curtain moment. After a few years of weights, I was starting to feel like I'd reached a plateau. I was not seeing changes to my body as often, nor was I going up in total weight. I felt a bit stuck. This was when I changed my whole mentality about lifting weights.

I read a few articles on it, and instead of trying to max out the weight now, I focus on the tempo, the squeeze and the movement of lifting lighter weights. I'm now doing one body part area per day, once a week. You may think that means that the area is neglected for the other 6 days, because we heal in 3 days. The reason why I do this now is so that I can really focus all of my intensity on one area, and give it my all.

My new thing is to do 3 different super set pairings for 3 sets each, with around 60 seconds rest in between each set. This gives me about 5 mins at the end of my workout to superset abs or calves (I switch these each day).

If you are really familiar with the split work-out now, you should try moving on to something like this. The key is to do relatively light weight as the reps are around 10-12. You should really feel burned out by the final superset. What's great about working out like this is that the variations are limitless with the tempo you lift the weights at. This is truly the next level of working out as you can hold your squat at the bottom for 2 seconds, or take 3 seconds going down on your bench each rep. You are messing with your body's time under tension and that makes it burn like crazy. This adds a number of new dimensions to the old movement of weight from point A to point B. It works conversely too, so instead of just pushing weight off of you at your normal speed, try exploding it off of you. This calls for my force and a greater demand on the muscles used, so they grow faster. Once you get into this, there is no going back.

It's also very important to start *carb cycling* when working out like this. Carb cycling simply means that on workout days you *eat starchy carbs like potatoes, sweet potatoes, brown rice, whole wheat pasta, nuts, whole grain bread etc*. And then on rest days, you avoid these types of carbs (but continue to eat your veggies).

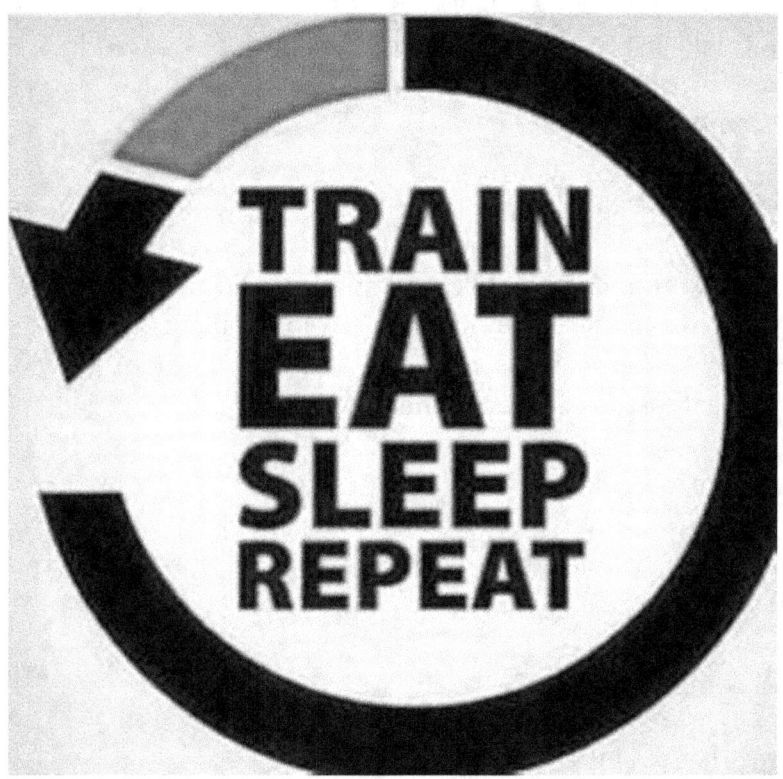

Tips for your Training Bible

If you ever get stuck in a rut with your progression, just get back to basics with your approach. Big people lift big, eat big protein and sleep long.

If you are trying to get big, you need to obviously eat more of the healthy food we talked about. Your muscle growth is the net of protein synthesis and protein breakdown. If you synthesize more than you naturally break-down (by just simply living), you will see gains. You want to keep your metabolism always moving so every 2-3 hours, hit it with some protein and veggies (pre made, small amounts of chicken and broccoli). It's crazy but eating more in this way, will make you thinner, and you'll never be hungry. If you can sustain this fuel injection schedule, you will see results very quickly. Your body will always be firing like a sports car and your work-outs will just be the finishing touches on your masterpiece.

Tips for dedicated lifters:

http://tinyurl.com/nu9jlaq

Here's your motivation. If you get down at the gym about pain, or feel like going home, just picture the guy from this video telling you that *it's still your motherf***ing set!* This video is a perfect proponent for why you should not eat fast food and only healthy.

http://tinyurl.com/pbjq3kh

And this is a great article for the holistic approach to working out and eating right:

http://tinyurl.com/mtk8yfb

Advanced Abs (6-8 Pack)

Alright, let's get down to brass tacks. No workout guide would be complete without a method for getting to that elusive 8-pack. You should know by now that it's really a by-product of a very lean diet. If you lose weight all over, you will expose the muscles in your midsection.

Let's be logical here. If you want that 8-pack, you need to shrink your stomach. You *cannot* let your belly get distended by big meals or bad food. That doesn't mean you have to eat 6 -7 small meals a day. Once you get your macros right, you can see that 1 single chicken breast with some sweet potatoes can cover a whole meal of calories. Go for small portions like that and snack on protein shakes.

But just like any other muscle group, if you train them with weight, they'll grow. Then, if you cut out the fat, the mirror may very well become *your new BFF*. You will have discovered *the Holy Grail* of working out.

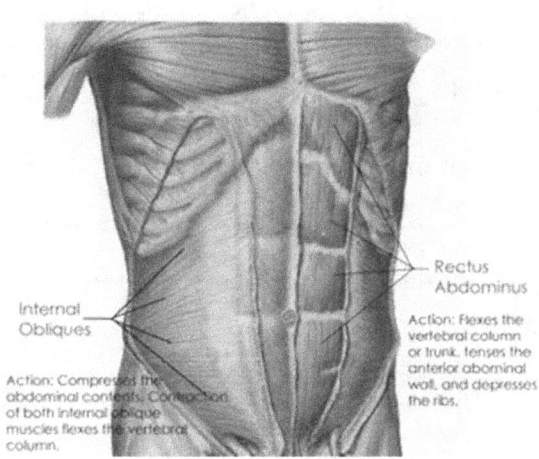

Think of your body as one big arm and your abs as the biceps. The methods that you use to make your bi's explode are the same methods you need for your abs. If you've been using your leg weight to do hanging leg raises then it's time to add a light dumbbell between your feet. If you can do dozens of crunches with relative ease, add a dumbbell or a plate to your chest.

One of the biggest errors we make in training abs is breathing. You need to *inhale deeply before executing the* movement and blow all of your air out *as you crunch or raise your legs.* This forces your abs to contract.

Now let's talk hanging leg raises. Try for 3 sets of 12-15 reps. These are really great for the *lower mid-section*. I like to vary how I raise my legs on these. On some I'll raise my legs to my waist, some above my head, some just bringing my knees up to my chest, and some turning to each side and bringing my knees up (hanging oblique knee raises). Keep your abs guessing.

Now for upper abs you want to do sit-ups on a decline bench. Try for 3 sets of 15-20 reps. Get an adjustable bench and put it in the decline position. You lie back and then lift up and again, mix it up. Do some straight sit-ups, bicycle crunches, reach for the ceiling sit-ups and medicine ball or weighted crunches.

For obliques I love grabbing the heaviest medicine ball, hugging it, and lifting myself up sideways on the 45 degree hyperextension bench. Try for 3 sets of 12-15 reps.

At this point it's key to make sure that you *DO NOT work abs every day* when you're going for the 8-pack.

Simply work them 2-3 times a week *heavy* and then give them time to rest. Keep them guessing all the time.

Physique athletes often have impressive abs so let's defer to them for advice:

http://tinyurl.com/pepff9n

Here are some other tips to think about when training the abs:

http://tinyurl.com/pfrlo54

Other Advanced Ab Exercises

Russian Twists (can be done with weights)

Flutter Kicks

Rope Cable Crunches

Ab Roll-Outs

Hanging Windshield Wipers – This is it. This exercise involves hanging from a bar, raising your legs up to your head, and then moving your legs back and forth like a windshield wiper down to waist level (if you go all the way down, you rest too much). They target about every muscle in your core and are a great exercise to shred away the last few inches covering your 8-pack. What's great is that you can do them anywhere. Even if you're at a park watching your kids, just grab a bar and go.

If you really want to get to the 8-pack, you have to be focused; you can't afford a day off or even an off day. If you hit a fat wall, then it is time to start using cardio and do that 5K run once a weekend. Count your macros, use weight on your ab workouts, don't drink alcohol, no cheat meals and you will get there my friend. We all have 8 packs in there somewhere.

These articles will get you pumped up for your 8-pack too:

http://tinyurl.com/ndocaq5

http://tinyurl.com/zern42d

And this article has methods for keeping your abs chiselled all year round. Wicked!

http://tinyurl.com/j8vgeb2

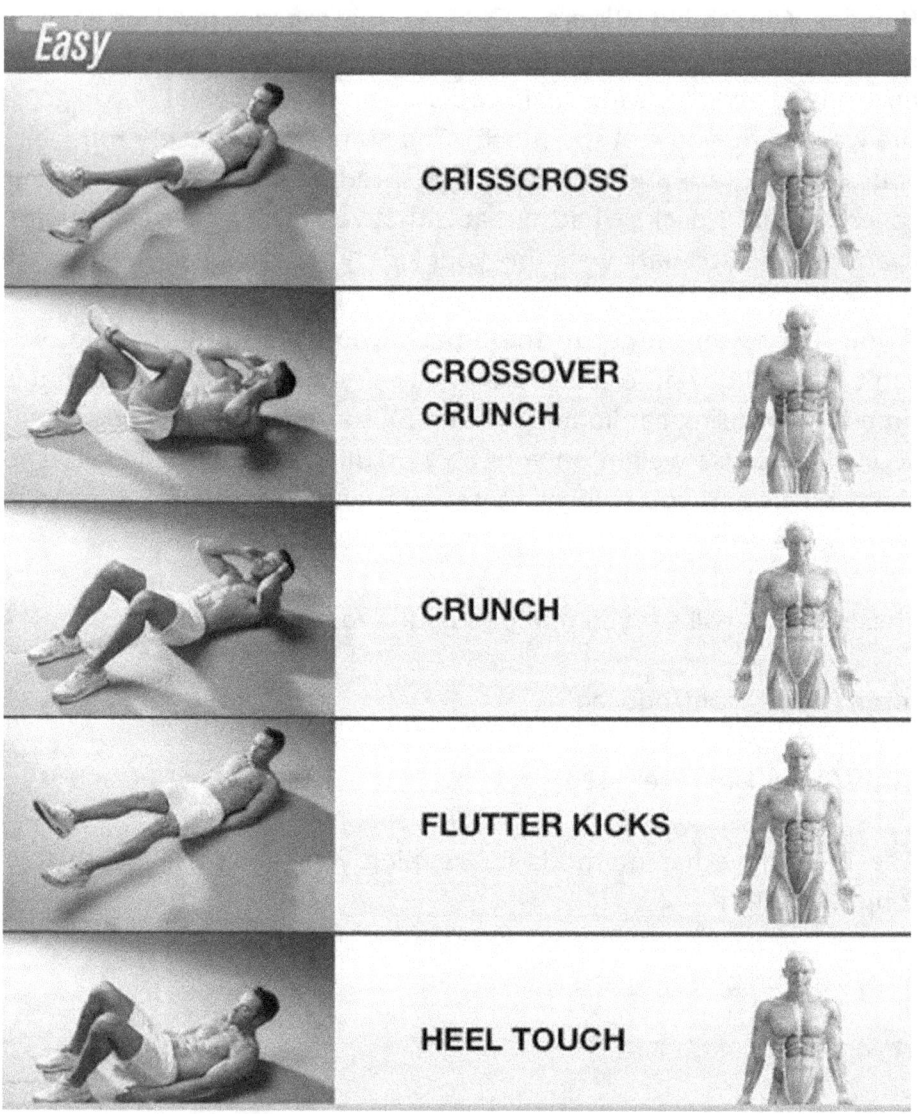

Easy

CRISSCROSS

CROSSOVER CRUNCH

CRUNCH

FLUTTER KICKS

HEEL TOUCH

Supplementation

So what's the deal with supplementation?

Is it cheating to ingest anything other than good, healthy food?

In my opinion, no, and it's not the same as doing 'roids. Do I recommend all of them? No. I think that most of them are truly snake oil and normally are purchased primarily because of hype.

Have I seen supplements get results? Hell yeah. Not taking supplements versus taking supplements is like riding a horse versus driving a high performance sports car. The latter is definitely more expensive than the first but it will get you there faster and you'll look goooood.

Besides your staple *whey protein* shake, here are some supplements I've tried and do recommend:

Casein Protein – This is similar to the normal protein shakes I keep banging on about but it takes longer to digest in comparison. Because of this, it keeps your body from being catabolic (destructive metabolism). I have this protein before I go to sleep so that my nightly fast and protein breakdown, is offset by steady muscle synthesis. You wake up in the morning feeling jacked. I definitely recommend this approach. It is also the ideal snack protein shake, or meal replacement, as it steadies you out for 3 hours if you need to skip a meal. When you look forward to your casein protein at night before your sleep, like a dessert, you're doing it right.

Creatine – Creatine is found naturally within our bodies and helps to supply energy to all cells. It increases the formation of ATP which is the currency of energy in our bodies and it *will* give you a quicker recovery along with an increase in muscle mass. Take it before your work-out in your pre shake. *Creatine monohydrate* is the one to go with. No studies have been done on it with kids under 18, so I don't recommend it – or any supplements – for kids.

This is a good article on creatine:

http://tinyurl.com/lg2szs

Glutamine – Glutamine is the most abundant amino acid in your body. Glutamine supplementation can reduce muscle breakdown and improve protein metabolism. I also take this in my post workout shake -- a heaping tablespoon of it. Powder is better than capsules for a lot of these supplements because you get more for your money. To get up to the amounts I needed for growth required taking 10 or more capsules every day. Sometimes this would trigger my gag reflex if I thought about it too much. Needless to say, I like powder.

This is a great article on glutamine:

http://tinyurl.com/l8yejxf

Caffeine -- Now you may be thinking, "*Is he talking about coffee*?" Kind of. Caffeine has terrific effects on fat loss by enhancing *lipolysis*. And because it's a stimulant, it gives you energy to perform your workouts. It's a *win/win* if you aren't near your bedtime. It should not be taken in excess, but it will definitely give you the pump you need to get going on those lethargic days. I get some caffeine from my *Optimum Nutrition Platinum PRE* shake before every workout.

Here's a good article about the benefits of caffeine:

http://tinyurl.com/25t27qz

If you want to see what hard core supplementation looks like, check out this video:

http://tinyurl.com/ht8sx2h

BCAA's – This is short for Branched Chain Amino Acids. They are made up of the essential aminos leucine, isoleucine and valine. Whereas the other amino acids we talked about are processed in the liver and gut, these go straight into the bloodstream and right to the muscles that need them. They are great for the hard core enthusiast looking to add muscle.

Fish Oil – I also take fish oil capsules every day. You can find these in the vitamin section at most supermarkets. I take this with my multivitamin each morning with my multi and Vitamin C. Fish oil is supposedly good for easing any pain in your joints caused by working out. It also has *omega-3* which is linked to preventing heart disease.

http://tinyurl.com/h3k7tpx

27

Anything Else?

I'm always searching for the perfect mix for my body. And I hope that you're now searching to do the same for yours. To that end, I'd like to recommend a few other online resources for encouragement and information:

http://cutandjacked.com/

https://www.facebook.com/Addicted2theGYMlife

https://www.facebook.com/AskKelechiOpara

https://www.facebook.com/LazarAngelovFitness

http://www.strengthsensei.com/charles-poliquin/

TC Luoma is one of my favourite fitness authors. Check out his pieces here:

http://tinyurl.com/j9q7tml

Arnold's Work-Out Plans (look at Part's 2, 3 and 4)
http://tinyurl.com/l4btt39

http://tinyurl.com/cph3ovq

Ronnie Coleman's Work-Out Plan

http://tinyurl.com/hxyl6ow

Kelechi Opara's Work-Out and Eating Plan

http://tinyurl.com/z8a9jgl

Alex Carneiro's Work-Out and Eating Plan

http://tinyurl.com/hfgjnkn

Why You Aren't Getting Big

http://tinyurl.com/j4oq3j6

Lazar Angelo's Work-Out and Eating Plan

http://tinyurl.com/zeqydm7

10 Mistakes Women Make In The Gym

http://tinyurl.com/mpeap4e

T-Nation Fat Loss Training Plan

http://tinyurl.com/ka8f65a

Bodybuilding.com Muscle Building Plan

http://tinyurl.com/ndyszr4

Build A Better Butt - For Women

http://tinyurl.com/pqqrhcs

The Jogging Delusion

http://tinyurl.com/jfbg2gm

Eating vs Working Out

http://tinyurl.com/j3noonh

Want Motivation To Change? John Burk Will Get You Off The Couch.

http://tinyurl.com/j63f9zv Hannibal For King - my idol

http://tinyurl.com/llqccvp

And the guy from my local gym is awesome. He will surely take over the fitness world. Jordan Metcalfe

http://www.ironplayground.com/

28

Advanced Eating

This section is for those who have been eating healthy for months and who work-out regularly. If you've been doing both, you should already be enjoying results. Congratulations!

You can now eat pretty much anything you want because your body will do a good job burning it off. Anything naughty that will keep you sane and loving life will stand as much chance in your body as a tab of butter in a hot pan. Just try to keep it mostly healthy and you'll be fine.

If you are looking to maintain a god body with a 6 or 8-pack, you still need to keep your eating strict (*unless you are some freak of nature, in which case, I'm jealous*).

To go to another extreme, there are some people who take their diets even further. I have a bodybuilding friend who eats a steak, nuts and an avocado each day for breakfast. The idea being that it keeps his testosterone pumping and sets him up for his five further meals of chicken and broccoli throughout the day. The dude is jacked. That's too hard core for me but to each their own.

Check out this fitness model's eating plan. It's pretty mental, but the results speak for themselves.

http://tinyurl.com/helanyf

Now feel free to open your diet to these foods:

Seafood! – *Tuna, salmon, sardines, trout.* Try bits of smoked salmon in your scrambled eggs. Yum. But stay away from shrimp and oysters (because of what they feed on).

Grains! – *Whole wheat bread, oatmeal, muesli, granola, brown rice*

Fruit! – Any of them, as long as they are fresh. Remember, *from the ground or a tree is good. Processed is bad.*

Nuts! – *Almonds, cashews, pistachios, walnuts, peanuts (peanut butter!)* Stay away from macadamia nuts and pecans, and be careful of trail mixes and dried fruits, as sometimes they have a really high fat content.

Everything in Moderation, Including Moderation

Cheat/Treat Meals

You will not become unhealthy from a single meal just like you will not become healthy from one meal. If you feel the need to splurge on some dessert, or beer or wine, you've now earned it. Having a treat every now and then will most likely help to keep you interested in eating and focused on eating healthy and it will keep you from craving bad foods. You can teach yourself how to act around temptations by giving in every now and then. It's a mostly psychological game that you are now prepared to play...and WIN!

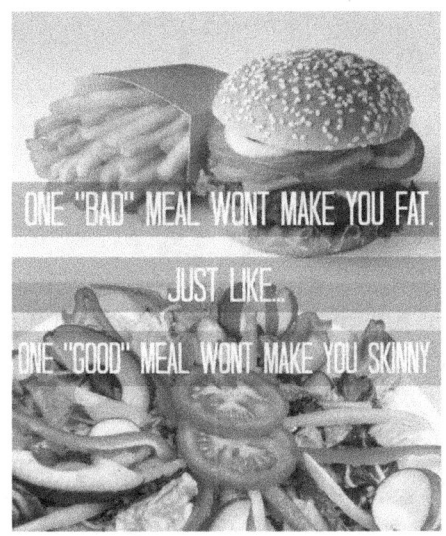

If you limit these splurges to *once a week* and to 1-2 meals, your body should process it fine (I still wouldn't suggest fast food).

Stick to eating and enjoying fresh food, even for cheat/treat meals!

29

Uncle Rudy's Tips

My books would not be complete without random thoughts that don't fit anywhere other than my head. Here's a few I've been saving for a rainy day...

Tip 1: Protein powder can help you out when you have no choice but to eat a low protein meal. So when you are out for dinner and there is nothing high protein on the menu, just remember to have a protein shake when you get home. The same way that eggs don't need to be cooked only one way, protein powder doesn't always need to be taken in a shake though. It can be put over cereal, yogurt, oatmeal etc. It's not how you get it in, it's all about getting it in.

Tip 2: If you are buying two steaks at a time, keep them stored in your fridge in a big plastic box that seals out air. This keeps them fresher for a few days. Nothing sucks more than letting good meat go bad.

Tip 3: Coffee, or the caffeine in it, is a great source of energy to get you through a workout and also contributes to fat loss.

Tip 4: I've come to find that with heavy lifting comes a bit of pain. Some is the normal wear and tear of DOMS (Delayed Onset Muscle Soreness) while some pain makes you really wonder if you have bone cancer or something. I sometimes feel this in my arms or legs after a workout. A great remedy for this pain is simply stretching while sitting or lying down. You'd be surprised how often your arms and legs are curled, whether it be sitting or at your desk typing.

Tip 5: I personally don't like the idea of too many unnatural movements with weights. Unnatural meaning not the up and down a muscle or joint is used to from life. Your knees and other joints are delicate in many ways. Subjecting them to stress they aren't used to (in the form of unnatural movements) is an easy way to get injured. I sometimes see people at the gym doing these backward curtsy movements where it is a lunge with one leg going behind the other one on the way down. To top it off, they do it with weight. Sure that may feel like a good butt blaster, but putting side pressure on your knee is an easy way to harm your ligaments. So forward lunges with weight are fine. Side lunges with weight are a no no from me.

Tip 6: Listen to your body. 6 days a week is probably the maximum anyone should be working out. But, if during this 6 day cycle, you have been going hard and your body needs a rest, take another day off. Heal up, recharge your batteries, and then go back the next day and kill it. Lack of rest is like spending too much time in the gym: Negative effects come a callin'.

Tip 7: The best time to look in the mirror is in the morning before you've had your eggs. Your nightly fast will leave your body cut up and tight. It's "abs"-olutely the best time to see results. Ouch.

Tip 8: Never shop for groceries when you're hungry. Hunger can *and will* bend your will towards trigger foods that ruin your plan and then ruin your body.

Tip 9: For further body changes, try changing your environment. Being hot and cold makes your body work harder, and burn more calories, to get back to homeostasis. If you get shipwrecked and you're on a raft, they tell you not to jump in the water even if it feels warmer. This is because water sucks the heat out of you. That's why swimming is such a great workout. You don't realize the amount of energy you are expending, just by acclimating to the water. So if you start to see a plateau, change your environment to make your body work a little harder.

Tip 10: Our adrenal glands secrete a hormone called cortisol, when we're stressed. It is bad for those who are pushing their bodies in the gym and need to stay stress free when they're resting. If we take 1,000 mgs of Vitamin C (usually one citrusy pill) when we're stressed, it decreases the amount of cortisol in our systems. A life hack here is that it works in any stressful situation. If you have stage fright, try a Vitamin C pill before speaking publicly and feel its calming results. You can find vitamin C supplements in almost every supermarket.

30

You're On Your Way

If you've made it this far, implemented the ideas and applied yourself diligently, **Good on Ya'!**

If you've just skipped to the end without reading any of it, well you're in luck too, because I sum it all up here.

It's overwhelming to try to change your eating, and work-out in one go. Split these two up. Lose weight first by eating healthy. Then and only then begin your work-outs.

Cooking your own meals is critical to understanding what you are putting into your body. You cannot trust other's food to be good for you. You must cook for yourself.

Macronutrients (protein, fat and carbs) are needed with every meal. Sugar is not a necessity in your daily meals because your insulin needs to be muted to encourage weight loss.

Fruit is sugar and prevents you from losing weight as it stimulates an insulin response.

Breakfast is critical to losing weight. It should consist mainly of eggs and can include healthy carbs if you like.

If you're trying to cut weight, lunch should contain fewer carbs than breakfast and dinner should be hardly any carbs at all.

Working out can easily be done at home with only your bodyweight for resistance.

Maximizing your lunch hour with a 45 minute workout gives you the perfect break in the day.

Consuming a protein shake before, a BCAA drink during, and a protein shake and food after your workout will maximize the results. Insulin needs to be exploited for muscle gains.

Weight training is better than cardio for keeping weight off.

In Conclusion And On To Volume 3

There is only one you. Why not be the best you? The self is an illusion, but your body is real. Why count the days when you can make the days count? You live in the most amazing period in human history. You have the most advanced knowledge at your fingertips on a machine in your pocket. We cannot hide behind ignorance any longer, especially when it comes to eating healthy. No one is going to look out for your health more than you. Trusting in soulless corporations will leave you hating your body. So give a damn. Look your best. Feel your best and kill with your new confidence. The world needs more winners and that is what a good body projects.

I'm just a regular guy with a regular job. If I can do it, then any of you can too.

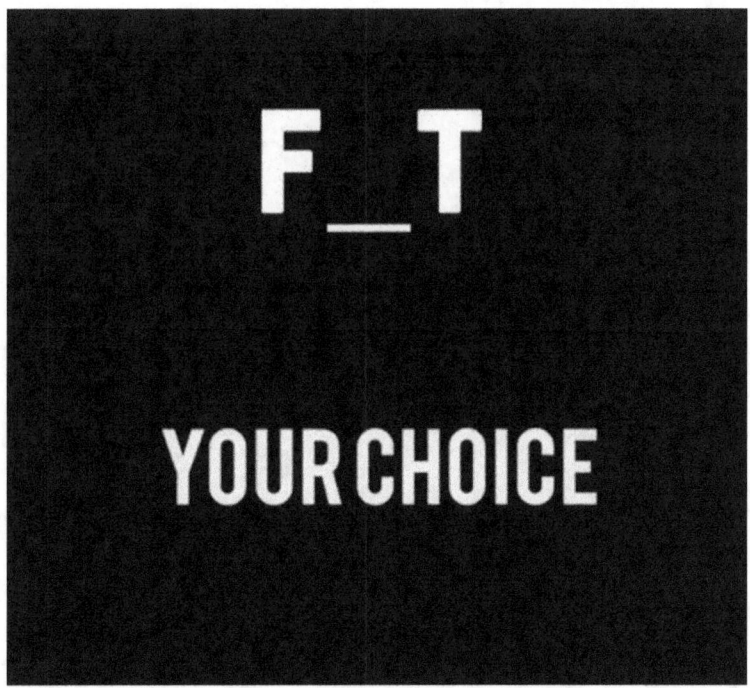

Table of Context